Biotechnology in Healthcare

Biotechnology in Healthcare

An introduction to biopharmaceuticals

Edited by

Gavin Brooks

BPharm, PhD, MRPharmS

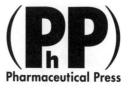

Pharmaceutical Press

Published by the Pharmaceutical Press
1 Lambeth High Street, London SE1 7JN

First published 1998

© 1998 Pharmaceutical Press

Cover design by Interbrand Newell & Sorrell, London
Text design by Barker/Hilsdon, Lyme Regis, Dorset
Typeset by Type Study, Scarborough, North Yorkshire
Printed in Great Britain by TJ International, Padstow, Cornwall

ISBN 0 85369 372 2

A catalogue record for this book is available from the British Library

For Anna

Contents

Preface

The powerful and extensive range of techniques that molecular biology now has to offer has enabled significant and rapid advances to be made in our understanding and treatment of a number of human diseases. Indeed, the recent upsurge in the number of small biotechnology companies wishing to capitalise on the plethora of research findings from academic institutions, for the purpose of developing novel approaches to drug discovery and development, illustrates the importance of molecular biology to the biopharmaceutical industry today. It is imperative, therefore, that all researchers and students involved in medical and scientific research and drug development have at least a basic understanding of the techniques of molecular biology and how they are being applied to the diagnosis and treatment of disease. This book is intended to serve as a source of information for medical, dental, pharmacy and science undergraduates and postgraduates and healthcare workers who wish to extend their knowledge of molecular biology and its clinical applications. The book is divided into discrete chapters, each of which addresses an individual area of biotechnology and describes the basics of that area followed by examples of how it is being used clinically and the relevance of the technique in healthcare today. The first three chapters provide a basic introduction to molecular biology, genetics and gene cloning, whereas subsequent chapters describe more specific techniques and applications of biotechnology, e.g. the polymerase chain reaction and DNA fingerprinting. It is hoped that this text will serve as a reference source for those healthcare workers who wish to extend their understanding of a variety of techniques that they will come across in their day-to-day duties and for any individual who is interested in learning more about recent developments in biotechnology and their relevance to the diagnosis of disease and clinical medicine.

Gavin Brooks
July 1998

Acknowledgements

I would like to take this opportunity to thank my co-authors, without whose contributions this volume would not have been possible. In addition, I would like to express my thanks to Paul Weller, John Wilson and other members of the Pharmaceutical Press for commissioning this book and for their help and support throughout the writing stages. Finally, I would like to thank my wife, Anna, and my parents for their constant support and encouragement during all stages of this project.

About the editor

Gavin Brooks obtained a first-class honours degree in pharmacy from the School of Pharmacy, University of London, in 1984 and subsequently registered as a pharmaceutical chemist in 1985. In October 1985, he was awarded a Royal Pharmaceutical Society Postgraduate Research Fellowship to enable him to undertake a PhD degree in the areas of organic chemistry and pharmacology at the School of Pharmacy, University of London. Dr Brooks then joined the Imperial Cancer Research Fund Laboratories in London as a post-doctoral fellow in 1988, where he investigated the signal transduction mechanisms involved in the progression of normal melanocytes to malignant melanoma cells. Following a successful period at the ICRF, Dr Brooks was recruited, in January 1992, to the Department of Cardiovascular Research, the Rayne Institute, St Thomas' Hospital, London, where he established an active cardiovascular cellular and molecular biology laboratory and rapidly became recognised as an expert in the area of cardiac myocyte cell cycle control. In July 1997, he joined Prolifix Ltd, a growing biopharmaceutical company interested in evaluating a range of novel therapeutic targets for the treatment of proliferative and infectious diseases. Recently, he accepted a lectureship position within the School of Animal and Microbial Sciences, University of Reading, where he is continuing his investigations to establish the role of the cell cycle in cardiovascular disease. Dr Brooks is the author of over 30 peer-reviewed original research papers and 18 review articles and currently lives in Henley-on-Thames with his wife, Anna, and their daughter, Katie.

Contributors

Sandra Amor BSc, PhD
Multiple Sclerosis Society Research Fellow, Department of
Neurodegenerative Disorders, Division of Neuroscience, Imperial
College School of Medicine, Charing Cross Hospital, Fulham Palace
Road, London W6 8RS

Colin D Bingle BSc, PhD
Lecturer in Respiratory Cell and Molecular Biology, Division of
Molecular and Genetic Medicine, University of Sheffield School of
Medicine, Sheffield S10 2RX

Gavin Brooks BPharm, PhD, MRPharmS
Lecturer in Biochemistry and Physiology, School of Animal and
Microbial Sciences, University of Reading, Whiteknights, PO Box 228,
Reading RG6 6AJ

Ian Gibson, BSc, PhD, MP
Dean of the School of Biological Sciences, University of East Anglia,
Norwich NR4 7TJ

Nicola Hardwick BSc
PhD Student, ICRF Oncology Group, The Hammersmith Hospital, 50
Du Cane Road, London W12 0HS

Vanessa Potter BSc, MB, ChB, MRCP
Clinical Research Fellow, CRC Department of Clinical Oncology,
University of Nottingham, City Hospital, Hucknall Road, Nottingham
NG5 1PB

Alastair D Reith BSc, PhD
Assistant Director, Molecular Neurobiology Research, Smithkline
Beecham Pharmaceuticals, New Frontiers Science Park North, Third
Avenue, Harlow CM19 5AW

Richard G Vile BSc, PhD
Molecular Medicine Program, Mayo Clinic, Rochester, Minnesota,
USA

Graham R Wallace BSc, PhD
Senior Research Fellow, Department of Ocular Immunology, The
Rayne Institute, St Thomas' Hospital, London SE1 7EH

Penella J Woll BMedSci, MB, BS, PhD, MRCP
Senior Lecturer and Consultant in Medical Oncology, CRC
Department of Clinical Oncology, University of Nottingham, City
Hospital, Hucknall Road, Nottingham NG5 1PB

1

An introduction to basic molecular biology

Gavin Brooks

The term 'molecular biology' covers a myriad of techniques and approaches that, nowadays, are used routinely in many scientific laboratories around the world. These techniques have been applied to research relating to almost every disease known to man, and it now is imperative that all researchers and students involved in medical and scientific research have at least a basic understanding of molecular biology and its terminology.

The aim of this opening chapter is to provide the reader with an introduction to the basic concepts and terminologies used in molecular biology. More specific and additional applications and aspects of molecular biology can be found in subsequent chapters.

DNA and RNA molecules

The basis of all molecular biology is the deoxyribonucleic acid (DNA) molecule. DNA is the most important substance known to man as it carries within its structure the hereditary information that determines the structures of proteins – the essential elements that make up cells and whole organisms. DNA also provides the instructions for directing cells to grow and divide and sends the messages required by fertilised eggs to differentiate into the multitude of specialised cells that make up our bodies. Since Watson and Crick first published the double helical structure of DNA in 1953, investigators have begun to understand more clearly how DNA controls the expression of genes and proteins within cells and consequently why one particular cell differentiates into one cell type, e.g. a brain cell, while another differentiates into a completely different cell type, e.g. a liver cell.

Chromosomes and chromatin

DNA is packaged within chromosomes in the nuclei of cells. Chromosomes are relatively large particles (a few micrometres in size) that are visible by light microscopy and are composed of a centromere from which protrudes four arms, each sealed by a telomere, which helps to confer stability to the ends of the chromosome. Essentially, these structures can be regarded as assemblies of units made up of DNA, ribonucleic acid (RNA) and proteins, which are precisely duplicated during cell division. The human somatic cell (i.e. any cell other than a gamete or germ cell precursor) contains 22 pairs of autosomal chromosomes and two sex-determining chromosomes – XX in the female and XY in the male. As somatic cells contain two copies of each chromosome they are referred to as diploid; germ cells, on the other hand, contain only one chromosome partner from each pair and are referred to as haploid. Chromosomes can become abnormal, e.g. as a result of the effects of certain drugs or other noxious agents, and this can lead to the development of diseases such as cancer and some cardiac myopathies. Such chromosomal abnormalities can be detected by molecular biological analyses, e.g. the polymerase chain reaction (Chapter 5), and often these approaches are used in the diagnosis of such disorders.

Chromosomes themselves consist of compactly folded mixtures of DNA and proteins called chromatin. Chromatin is composed of an approximately 1-m-long, 0.2-nm-thick string of DNA wound around a core of proteins called histones. Chromatin itself is composed of individually packaged units called nucleosomes which, by electron microscopy, appear as beads on a thin string. The human genome consists of approximately 3×10^7 nucleosomes, each of which measures about 11 nm in diameter. Each nucleosome consists of two copies of four different histones, H2A, H2B, H3 and H4, around which is wound a constant length of DNA. Each nucleosome is separated from its neighbours by a length of DNA that is bound to a fifth histone protein called H1. Thus, although the core histone components of each nucleosome remain constant in each repeated unit, different sequences of DNA are wrapped around them. In this way, the cell can package very large amounts of DNA into a very small volume. In addition to histones, DNA also is covered with other proteins within the chromosome, including transcription factors, other structural proteins and various regulatory factors such as nuclear receptors, e.g. steroid receptors.

Base pairing

The DNA molecule is a double-stranded helix composed of two single-stranded monomers. Each strand is made up of nucleotides composed of a phosphosugar component attached to one of four different bases: the two purines, adenine (A) and guanine (G); and the two pyrimidines, thymine (T) and cytosine (C). Each nucleotide is linked to its neighbours via covalent bonds made between the phosphates and sugars, forming a sugar–phosphate backbone. Each base has a specific, high affinity for only one other base such that G recognises (base pairs with) C and A base pairs with T. The number of base pairs in a particular DNA sequence is used to record the size of that sequence, e.g. the human insulin gene is approximately 1.5 thousand base pairs (kilobase pairs, kb), whereas the human dystrophin gene is more than 2000 kb. The two strands of DNA are held together by non-covalent hydrogen bonding between the bases on each strand. As base pairing is very specific, the nucleotide sequence of one strand can be deduced from, and is determined by, the other strand. Each strand of double-stranded helical DNA is directional such that each has a 5′ and 3′ end; thus, the two strands are said to be complementary and antiparallel to one another (Figure 1.1). When a new DNA molecule is synthesised, synthesis always occurs

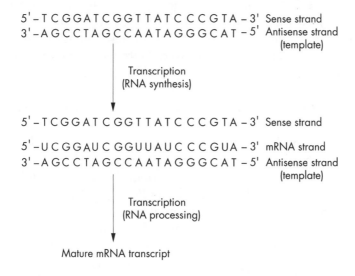

Figure 1.1   Schematic diagram to show the process of transcription of a hypothetical gene located in a double-stranded DNA sequence.

in a 5′ to 3′ direction. Thus, the synthesis of the two strands of DNA occurs in opposite directions since the 5′ end of one strand is base paired with the 3′ end of the other (Figure 1.1).

Transcription

One of the two strands of DNA is called the coding or sense strand and is identical to a messenger RNA molecule, which is an intermediate product between DNA and protein. The DNA sequence that is copied into an mRNA molecule is called a gene. Other RNA molecules are also produced from DNA and are used directly in the cell, e.g. transfer RNA and ribosomal RNA. Not all DNA codes for RNA; in fact, the majority of the DNA in the genome does not code for anything specific and is called silent or nonsense DNA. Nonsense DNA is important, however, for separating gene sequences from each other (if individual genes were not separated in this way, problems could occur for the cell when it had to decide which protein to make, as specific recognition sequences (see below) found upstream of the transcribed gene would be lost in an adjacent gene sequence). The DNA strand that is antiparallel to the coding strand is called the non-coding or antisense strand. By convention, the coding strand and mRNA strand are written from left to right, corresponding to the 5′ to 3′ direction. When a new protein is required by the cell, a portion of the coding strand of DNA is copied into a single-stranded RNA molecule by a process known as transcription, which relies on complementarity of base pairing between DNA bases and RNA bases. The nucleotide sequence that is copied into RNA specifies an amino acid sequence from which a protein is ultimately produced by a process called translation. RNA is made up of four different purine or pyrimidine bases on a phosphosugar backbone. Three of these bases are identical to those found in DNA, namely A, G and C, whereas T is replaced by uridine (U) in RNA, in which it base pairs with A (U is identical to T except that it does not have a methyl group on the basic ring). The cell can synthesise different types of RNA, including messenger RNA (mRNA), which corresponds to a nucleotide sequence that specifies an amino acid sequence; ribosomal RNA (rRNA), which is the most abundant form of RNA and is important in protein synthesis; and transfer RNA (tRNA), which is involved in transporting amino acids to the site of translation.

The process of RNA transcription proceeds as follows: RNA is transcribed from the non-coding strand of DNA (also referred to as the DNA template) and is synthesised in a 5′ to 3′ direction from the coding strand of DNA. Transcription of mRNA begins when the enzyme called RNA polymerase II recognises a specific sequence in the non-coding strand (called the initiation sequence), enabling it to bind to the 3′ end of the non-coding DNA strand. This attachment of RNA polymerase II is accompanied by a substantial conformational change in the DNA, resulting in a local opening of the DNA duplex to enable the RNA molecule to be copied from the DNA template. Nucleotides are then recruited to the region, and those complementary to the template are linked together to produce a new mRNA molecule that is complementary to the non-coding strand and identical to the coding strand of DNA since its sequence has been determined by the base pairing of As to Us and Cs to Gs. Similarly, just as the DNA template contains specific sequences that instruct RNA polymerase II to initiate transcription, so there are other sequences that instruct the enzyme to terminate the process such that the enzyme will be found at the 5′ end of the non-coding strand at the end of transcription. Once transcribed, the mRNA molecule is further processed in the nucleus by various splicing enzymes since not all of the copied mRNA molecule will code for a protein. The coding portion of the gene is located on one or more sections of the gene called exons (since these sections *ex*it the nucleus into the cytoplasm). The regions located between the exons do not code for protein and are called introns (since they remain *in*side the nucleus). The introns are excised from the mRNA molecule by forming loops called lariats which are then degraded in the nucleus. The 5′ and 3′ ends of the exon(s) also are not always coding sequences even though they form part of the mature mRNA molecule. Thus, the 5′ end of the exon becomes blocked by a 5′ to 5′ sugar–phosphate covalent bond called the RNA cap, whereas the 3′ end of the exon has a string of repetitive As attached, which is known as the poly(A) tail. Indeed, mRNA is commonly referred to as poly(A)-rich RNA. Once processed in this manner, the mature mRNA molecule is transported into the cytoplasm of the cell, where it is translated into protein (Figure 1.2).

Translation

Within each mature mRNA molecule, groups of three consecutive nucleotides form codons, each codon of which ultimately specifies one amino acid, e.g. the codon AUG encodes for methionine. It is the codons that form what is known as the genetic code and, as there are four nucleotides, there are 4^3 (64) possible codons. However, since only 20 amino acids are known, some amino acids are specified by more than one codon. In the process of translation, specific codons are recognised

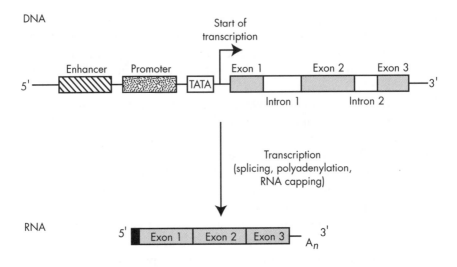

Figure 1.2 Hypothetical structure of a gene showing possible positions of enhancer, promoter, TATA box, exons and introns and subsequently how the mRNA molecule is modified prior to translation in the cytosol.

by tRNA molecules, each of which carries a specific amino acid and attaches this to the corresponding sequence on the mRNA molecule. Thus, the amino acid chain grows as directed by the codon sequence on the mRNA molecule. The translation process occurs on the ribosomes, which bind the mRNA, tRNA, rRNA and ribosomal proteins together in a complex that allows the mRNA code to be read and translated into a polypeptide chain. Synthesis of the amino acid chain begins with the amino-terminal amino acid and finishes with the carboxy-terminal amino acid and is encoded by the DNA coding sequence when read in the 5′ to 3′ direction. Three of the 64 possible RNA codon combinations do not code for a specific amino acid. Instead, these three codons (UAA, UGA and UAG) serve as termination signals for protein synthesis. Hence, once this codon is reached the newly synthesised protein will dissociate from the ribosomal complex and begin its function in the cell. In addition to the three termination codons, the AUG sequence (which encodes the amino acid methionine) can act as an initiation sequence for translation. Obviously, many possible methionines will be encoded within any particular protein, and other sequences that are 5′ (upstream) of the actual initiation AUG sequence play a pivotal role in determining exactly which methionine residue will initiate protein synthesis.

Complementary DNA (cDNA)

One of the most commonly used terms in molecular biology is cDNA, which is a double-stranded complementary DNA copy of a single-stranded mRNA molecule synthesised *in vitro* by reverse transcription. The mechanism of reverse transcription is described in detail in Chapter 5, but, in brief, it involves a three-step process. In the first step, a strand of DNA that is complementary to the mRNA strand is synthesised using the enzyme reverse transcriptase and an oligodeoxythymidine primer that binds to the poly(A) tail of the mRNA sequence. In the next step, the mRNA strands of the mRNA–DNA hybrid are destroyed using the enzyme RNase H. The final step involves generating a DNA copy of the single-stranded DNA that was left following degradation of the mRNA strand. The final double-stranded DNA molecule is known as cDNA and represents a genetic sequence that lacks any introns. Thus, cDNAs are used routinely in cloning experiments when high expression of a particular gene product is required (Chapter 3).

Regulation of gene expression

Of the 2×10^9 base pairs that constitute the human genome, the majority are never transcribed into RNA. However, certain regions of the non-transcribed DNA have specific functions that instruct the cell to transcribe a specific gene. For example, RNA polymerases are instructed to attach to a short DNA sequence called the promoter that is upstream (5′) of the gene of interest (Figure 1.2). Although the promoter site is essential for instructing RNA polymerase where to start RNA synthesis, it is not sufficient by itself to permit the process to occur; other DNA sequences also are required. These additional DNA sequences are called enhancers and they recognise specific protein factors in the cell, e.g. transcription factors (Figure 1.2). A factor that binds an enhancer is said to regulate gene transcription in a *trans*-regulatory manner and is referred to as a *trans*-activating factor, i.e. it is a protein produced from a gene that is physically distinct from the regulated gene, e.g. on a different chromosome. In contrast, the enhancer regulates gene transcription in a *cis*-regulating manner following the binding of a specific *trans*-activating protein. Activation of an enhancer results in an up to 1000-fold increase in the basal rate of transcription. Indeed, the effect of an enhancer on the rate of transcription is so strong that the effects still can be observed if it is placed at a distance several thousand base pairs from the transcription start site. Furthermore, enhancers are able to function in either orientation and therefore do not necessarily need to reside 5′ to a gene – they can be located within, or even downstream from, the transcribed region.

DNA sequences that are recognised by specific factors are commonly referred to as responsive elements, and all have regions, called consensus sequences, that are recognised by specific proteins. Thus, a consensus sequence is one that represents the bases found most often at each position when a large number of similar DNA sequences are compared. Two common consensus sequences are the TATA box, which consists of seven nucleotides, five of which are invariant, and the CAAT box, which also contains invariant and variant nucleotides. Different enhancers have consensus sequences that are different for different regulatory proteins, e.g. the glucocorticoid responsive element (GRE) has a consensus sequence that is different from the cyclic AMP responsive element (CRE), although a core consensus sequence for all eukaryotic enhancers has been identified as 5′-GTGAAG-3′.

Analysis of DNA

Probably the most basic of all procedures in molecular biology is the purification of nucleic acid. Many different approaches can be used to study DNA, and it is impossible to give an exhaustive list of all available methodologies here. However, a few of the routine procedures used are detailed below.

Preparation and purification of DNA

DNA is a double-stranded molecule that is extremely stable. The stability of DNA can be demonstrated by the ability to extract and purify this molecule from archival and even mummified remains that could be thousands of years old. The key step in isolating DNA is the removal of proteins, which can be achieved by the sequential extraction of aqueous solutions of nucleic acids with phenol, then phenol/chloroform and finally with chloroform alone. DNA then is recovered from the extracted aqueous solution by precipitation with ethanol. Although this procedure produces good-quality DNA from cDNA preparations necessary for cloning, additional measures are required for preparation of DNA from cells and/or tissues. In this case, most of the protein is removed by digestion with proteolytic enzymes such as pronase or proteinase K prior to extraction with organic solvents. The above methods can be used to isolate

DNA sequences that are >30 kb in length, although more commonly sequences of 10–30 kb are recovered.

Once isolated, the DNA preparation can be further purified by resuspending the precipitated DNA pellet in distilled water and reprecipitating with ethanol, by chromatography through Sephadex G-50, which separates high-molecular weight DNA from smaller molecules, or by agarose gel electrophoresis. Although these techniques will not be discussed further here, details can be found in the texts listed in the Further reading section at the end of this chapter.

Detection of specific DNA sequences

Two of the most commonly used techniques for determining the presence of a specific DNA sequence or gene in a preparation of genomic DNA are Southern blotting and the polymerase chain reaction (PCR).

Southern blotting (Figure 1.3)

This method, which was first developed by Edward Southern in 1975, takes advantage of the fact that DNA fragments of different sizes can be separated in an electric field by agarose gel electrophoresis. The separated DNA fragments then are denatured within the gel in the presence of alkali, neutralised and then transferred and immobilised onto a nitrocellulose or nylon filter. The DNA attached to the filter then is incubated (hybridised) to a ^{32}P-labelled cDNA or RNA probe that carries the sequence of the gene of interest. If the gene of interest is expressed in the immobilised DNA sample, the radiolabelled probe will bind to it in a specific manner and this binding can be observed as an image on photographic film following autoradiography. This technique has become the standard method for locating specific sequences in cloned DNA and also for identifying sequences within digests of total eukaryotic DNA.

Polymerase chain reaction (PCR)

Over the past few years, PCR has become a routine method for amplifying specific sequences of DNA either in a cloned cDNA fragment or in a total DNA preparation (see Chapter 5 for full details). One advantage of PCR over other methods of DNA purification and separation is that the reaction can be carried out on total DNA that has not had to be fragmented with restriction enzymes (these are endonucleases, isolated

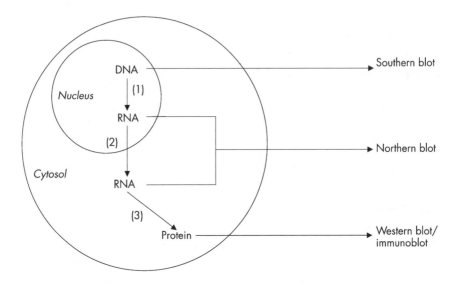

Figure 1.3   Schematic diagram to show where the processes of RNA synthesis (1), RNA processing (2) and translation (3) occur within a cell and the techniques used to identify DNA, RNA and protein species within a cell.

primarily from prokaryotes, that recognise specific sequences within double-stranded DNA and are used to 'cut' DNA into different sized fragments. There are a number of known restriction enzymes, each of which recognises a different sequence, and different stretches of DNA will produce different fragmentation patterns when cut with these enzymes since each sequence is unique. The different fragments then can be separated and visualised by agarose gel electrophoresis. Once the DNA fragment of interest has been amplified, it is separated on an agarose gel and subjected to Southern blotting as described above.

Analysis of RNA

Preparation and purification of mRNA

Unlike DNA, which is a relatively stable molecule, mRNA is rapidly degraded after death and has a very short half-life once extracted from cells or tissues. One of the major reasons for this is contamination by

RNases – a ubiquitous series of heat-stable enzymes that rapidly degrade RNA. These enzymes are present in blood, all tissues, most bacteria and moulds that are present in the environment and even on the fingertips of investigators. Therefore, any analysis of RNA needs to be carried out under very clean conditions and all operators should wear gloves. Since mRNA represents only 2–3% of all RNA species in a cell, some additional purification is required before analysis. One common method for the preparation of total RNA involves rapid homogenisation of fresh or rapidly frozen material in guanidinium thiocyanate, which inactivates RNases, followed by extraction with phenol/chloroform and precipitation of the extracted RNA with ethanol as described for DNA above. The RNA pellet then is extracted with a high concentration of salt, which solubilises double-stranded nucleic acids (the remaining traces of DNA and small RNAs) but not single-stranded rRNA or mRNA. The yield of total RNA by this method is in the region of 1 μg of total RNA per mg of fresh tissue, although this does depend upon the cell/tissue type under investigation. If the gene of interest is not expressed at particularly high levels it may be necessary to purify this preparation still further to enrich for mRNA species. There are many commercial kits now available that make the preparation of mRNA relatively simple. Most are based on the principle that mRNA has a poly(A) tail (see above) and that, in the presence of salt, hydrogen bonds will form readily between synthetic homopolymers of either uridine [poly(U)] or thymidine [oligo(dT)], i.e. those bases that base pair specifically with A. When the salt is removed, the hydrogen bonds dissociate, thereby enabling the bound mRNA to be separated from the synthetic oligonucleotide. When oligo(dT) is immobilised on a solid support and mixed with total RNA, the poly(A) tail of the mRNA component will hybridise to the oligo(dT) in the presence of high salt, whereas the rRNA is washed away. Rewashing the oligo(dT)–mRNA hybrid with water then releases an enriched mRNA preparation that can be precipitated with ethanol and the pellet resuspended in water before analysis.

Detection of specific RNA sequences

As with the detection of DNA, a number of different techniques are available for the detection of mRNA levels within a sample. These techniques include Northern blotting and reverse transcription–PCR.

Northern blotting (Figure 1.3)

This is a similar technique to Southern blotting above. Briefly, it is a method of separating an RNA sample according to size in a denaturing agarose gel followed by transfer and immobilisation of the denatured RNA onto a nitrocellulose or nylon filter. The filter then is used in a hybridisation assay with a radiolabelled cDNA probe that is specific for a selected gene. Quantitation of mRNA expression is carried out by autoradiography followed by densitometry of the resultant photographic signal(s).

Reverse transcription–PCR

This method is described in detail in Chapter 5 and is used routinely to monitor changes in mRNA expression of a particular gene following, for example, treatment of cells with a drug. Although the method can be used to quantitate levels of mRNA expression in a particular situation, it is important that a number of controls are included in the analysis. Indeed, Northern blotting remains the preferred technique for quantitating levels of expression of a particular mRNA species.

Analysis of proteins

Preparation and purification of proteins

Proteins can be isolated from cells or tissues by a number of procedures. Initial disruption of the cells is achieved by osmotic shock, ultrasonic vibration, grinding or lysis in a detergent-containing buffer. It is important, however, to include a range of protease inhibitors in any buffers since, once the cell is disrupted, a number of proteases will be released into the milieu and could break down a number of labile proteins that normally would be separated from these degradative enzymes. These procedures dissociate most cellular membranes, including plasma membranes and those of the endoplasmic reticulum. This then is followed by fractionation into the various subcellular components of the cell, which can be achieved by either filtration, chromatography or centrifugation. These steps enable separation of contaminating nucleic acids, mitochondria and lysosomes from the protein preparation. Further purification of some proteins that are heat stable (approximately 5% of all cellular proteins) can be achieved by boiling the protein extract for approximately 5 minutes, followed by centrifugation, which will pellet the heat-labile proteins in the sample. Once the protein extract has been purified in this manner, it can be analysed for the presence of specific proteins by one of the following methods.

Detection of specific proteins

A variety of detection methods are available for determining the presence of specific proteins in an extract, most of which rely upon the interaction of the protein with a specific antibody (see Chapter 11 for further details regarding protein–antibody interactions). Although it is possible to visualise certain proteins on a polyacrylamide gel by staining the separated proteins with Coomassie blue or silver stain, these approaches do not provide direct evidence for the presence of a specific protein – an antibody would be required to demonstrate the presence of the protein.

Polyacrylamide gel electrophoresis and immunoblotting (Western blotting) (Figure 1.3)

This method is one of the most commonly used analytical techniques for demonstrating the presence of a particular protein in a sample preparation. The method relies on the fact that proteins usually have a net positive or negative charge that reflects the mixture of charged amino acids that they contain. If an electric field is applied to a solution containing a protein molecule, the protein will migrate at a rate that depends upon its net charge and on its size and shape (electrophoresis). A modified version of this separation developed in the mid-1960s, called sodium dodecylsulphate polyacrylamide gel electrophoresis (SDS-PAGE), uses a highly cross-linked gel of polyacrylamide, as an inert matrix through which the proteins migrate, and the detergent, SDS. The SDS is negatively charged and large numbers of SDS molecules are bound by each protein molecule, which tends to overcome the intrinsic charge of the protein, ensuring that each protein migrates towards the positive electrode when a current is applied. Proteins of the same size then tend to behave similarly and larger molecules are retarded much more than smaller ones as the polyacrylamide acts as a molecular sieve. As a result, a complex mixture of proteins is fractionated into a series of discrete protein bands arranged in order of their molecular weight. SDS-PAGE is therefore a very powerful procedure for analysing and separating proteins and can be used to analyse all types of proteins, including those that are water insoluble.

The method is capable of separating around 50 different proteins from a complex mixture of proteins although other techniques, e.g. two-dimensional electrophoresis, are capable of separating more than 1000 proteins on a single gel.

In the immunoblotting procedure, a protein mixture is separated into proteins of different size by SDS-PAGE. The resolved proteins are then transferred to a nitrocellulose filter and incubated with an antibody that specifically recognises the protein of interest. A secondary antibody that is either attached to an enzyme such as horseradish peroxidase or labelled with a radioactive isotope, e.g ^{125}I, that recognises the first antibody is then incubated with the filter. When the substrate for the enzyme is subsequently incubated with the filter, a colour reaction will develop specifically in the region of the protein of interest and can be visualised either directly or as an image on photographic film (in the case of radiolabelled secondary antibodies this image is visualised directly without the need for a substrate). The levels of protein expression can then be determined by densitometry.

Immunoprecipitation

In this technique, the protein of interest is precipitated from a mixture of proteins by first incubating with an antibody that is specific for the protein of interest (primary antibody). A secondary antibody that recognises an immunoglobulin component of the primary antibody is then added to the mix. This secondary antibody is covalently linked to Sepharose or agarose beads, making it possible to isolate the protein of interest by centrifugation as a complex comprising the protein of interest, the primary antibody and the secondary antibody attached to Sepharose beads. The immunoprecipitate can then be separated by SDS-PAGE, which will release the isolated protein from the complex. The isolated protein can then be identified with the same primary antibody by Western blotting or the nitrocellulose filter could be incubated with an antibody directed against another protein to determine whether the first protein exists as a complex with another protein *in vivo*.

Immunocytochemistry

This technique enables the investigator to determine the expression and localisation of a particular protein in a tissue section. A thin section (a few micrometres thick) of the tissue of interest is prepared and incubated with the primary antibody. Following detection of the primary antibody with an appropriate fluorescence-labelled secondary antibody, the expression and localisation of the protein of interest can be observed by fluorescence microscopy.

Conclusions and summary

This chapter has described the basic concepts of DNA and RNA structure, transcription and translation and the procedures for purifying and identifying specific sequences or proteins in a nucleic acid or protein preparation. It is essential that any undergraduate or postgraduate investigator wishing to use molecular biology techniques understands the basic principles involved in these procedures before fully exploiting the potential of these exciting technologies.

Further reading

Alberts A, Bray D, Lewis J, *et al.*, eds (1994) *Molecular Biology of the Cell*, 3rd edn. New York: Garland Publishing.

Kendrew J, ed. (1994) *The Encyclopedia of Molecular Biology*. Oxford: Blackwell Science.

Sambrook J, Fritsch E F, Maniatis T (1989) *Molecular Cloning. A Laboratory Manual*, 2nd edn. Cold Spring Harbor, NY: Cold Spring Harbor Laboratory Press.

Swynghedauw B, Barrieux A (1993) Molecular biology for cardiologists: a teaching article (part 1). *Cardiovasc Res* 27: 2–8.

Swynghedauw B, Moalic J-M, Bourgeois F, Barrieux A (1993) An introduction to the jargon of molecular biology: a teaching article (part 2). *Cardiovasc Res* 27: 1566–1575.

Watson J D, Tooze J, Kurtz D T, eds (1983) *Recombinant DNA. A Short Course*. New York: Scientific American Books.

2

Molecular genetic mapping of disease genes

Alastair D Reith

An intuitive understanding of a hereditary basis of disease has been appreciated in distinct societies over many centuries, but it was not until the rediscovery of the work of Mendel in the early 1900s that genetics became established as a scientific discipline. As discussed in Chapter 1, chromosomes are the subcellular structures that bear genetic information. Initially there was considerable debate as to whether the genetic information resided in the DNA or protein components of chromosomes, and it was not until the structure of the DNA double helix was solved in 1953 that the molecular basis of heredity became apparent. Rapid progress has been made subsequently in our understanding of how information represented by the sequence of nucleotide bases within a gene is faithfully converted to encode proteins, the normal functioning of which is necessary for normal development and homeostasis (Chapter 1).

Given this flow of genetic information, it is apparent that changes in nucleotide sequence of polypeptide coding regions and gene regulatory elements can alter the expression and function of specific proteins. In many instances, such variation has no deleterious effect and contributes to genetic diversity within the gene pool of an outbreeding population. However, some nucleotide changes in certain genes constitute deleterious mutations (genotypic changes) that manifest as an inherited disease or susceptibility to particular conditions (phenotypic changes).

Only in a very small number of genetic diseases is there any pre-existing knowledge of the enzymatic defect responsible. The power of approaches to identify gene(s) responsible for a given hereditary condition lies in there being no absolute requirement of prior knowledge of the mechanism of disease progression. In addition, gene mapping methodologies are entirely generic and can be applied to any trait for which a genetic contribution can be established.

Genetic disorders can be categorised to three types, each of which presents differing challenges in understanding their molecular basis. Single-gene disorders are conferred by mutation of a single gene and include conditions such as cystic fibrosis, β-thalassaemia, Huntington's disease and myotonic dystrophy. In contrast, complex or polygenic disease traits result from the combinatorial effects of several genes, mutations in each of which contribute to the disease phenotype. A further elaboration is seen in multifactorial disorders, in which disease results from mutations in several disease susceptibility genes that act together with environmental factors.

Here, I discuss some of the molecular genetic technologies that underpin current efforts to identify disease susceptibility genes. As single-gene disorders are more amenable to genetic analysis, these have provided a focus in development of the necessary technologies for cloning disease gene loci. More recent developments, particularly in the area of the Human Genome Project, are now facilitating the identification of genes that contribute to complex genetic diseases. These include many common conditions, such as heart disease, rheumatoid arthritis, various cancers, multiple sclerosis, schizophrenia, autism, manic depression, alcoholism, diabetes and asthma, that create major demands on healthcare budgets. Knowledge of specific gene defects enables the development of screening procedures to distinguish unaffected and susceptible individuals. Furthermore, analysis of the range of molecular lesions that confer disease phenotypes provides a first step in understanding the molecular mechanism of a genetic disease and can form a basis for the design and development of potential therapeutic strategies.

Mendelian inheritance and recombination

In humans, most cells are diploid, in that they carry two copies of each of the autosomal chromosomes (23 in humans) plus the sex chromosomes X and Y. One copy of each of the autosomal chromosomes is inherited from each parent, together with a maternal X chromosome and an X or Y paternal chromosome. During normal cell division, each chromosome pair is duplicated and segregates appropriately such that both daughter cells carry the same diploid set of chromosomes.

Single-gene defects generally exhibit fairly simple patterns of inheritance, said to be Mendelian. Autosomal gene mutations can be dominant, where the disease phenotype arises as a consequence of mutation of one gene copy (allele), or recessive, in which case both alleles of the gene must be mutated to result in disease. Dominant mutations that have high penetrance tend to be selected against within an outbreeding population. However, in cases of late onset of disease, or variable penetrance, off-spring may be produced each of which would have 50% probability of inheriting the dominant mutant trait. By way of contrast, individuals bearing one copy of a recessive mutation are phenotypically normal, despite the presence of a single mutant allele, but can pass the mutation to their offspring. Offspring of such a 'carrier' and an individual bearing both normal copies of this gene have a 50% probability of also being carriers, but once again no disease would be apparent. In contrast, offspring of two carriers would have a 50% chance of being carriers but in addition a 25% chance of inheriting both mutant alleles. It is these individuals that would be expected to develop the inherited disease.

In contrast to normal diploid cells, gametes (egg and sperm) are haploid in that they each carry only a single copy of each autosome, plus X or Y. The process by which a haploid genome is generated from the normal diploid genome is termed meiosis. An important feature of meiosis is that it also provides an opportunity for reciprocal exchange of genetic information between maternal and paternal chromosomes (Figure 2.1). The ability of chromatid pairs to recombine at meiosis results in reshuffling of genes inherited from each, so promoting diversity in the genetic information transmitted to the subsequent generation. Recombination also lies at the heart of efforts to map and clone disease genes. In principle, two loci that lie close together on a chromosome have a high probability of being inherited together and hence show tight linkage. The further the distance between the two loci, the greater the probability of a recombination event separating them, so revealing a lower probability of linkage. The recombination frequency observed between two linked markers is a genetic distance measured in centi-morgans (cM), named after the early geneticist T H Morgan, with a recombination frequency of 1% being equivalent to 1 cM.

Mapping the human genome

In general terms, disease gene identification proceeds through a series of steps, outlined in Figure 2.2. First, to establish a Mendelian inheritance of a given disease, it is necessary to have access to detailed information of large family pedigrees. With such resources at hand, the chromosomal location of the disease gene can be defined by correlating disease occur-rence with inheritance of markers, the chromosomal location of which has been defined previously. It follows that the more detailed the set of

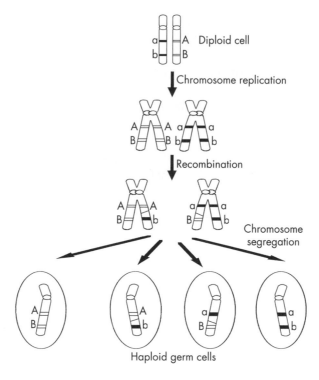

Figure 2.1 Genetic recombination. Germ cell production requires a reduction in the normal diploid chromosome complement to a haploid genome by the process of meiosis. This also provides an opportunity for recombination between paternal and maternal chromosomes. Following replication, sister chromatids of homologous chromosomes may align and a reciprocal exchange of genetic information can occur. In this case, recombination generates germ cells carrying each parental gene combination (ab or AB) as well as novel combinations Ab and aB. Recombination promotes genetic diversity between generations. The recombination frequency observed between genes A/a and B/b also provides a basis for genetic mapping of chromosomal markers.

known genetic markers accurately mapped to the human genome, the easier disease gene mapping becomes. Having defined a minimal chromosomal fragment, DNA clones of this region are sought. Large-scale physical mapping efforts are under way to provide resources of human DNA clones of specified regions of chromosomes. Analysis of these genomic clones identifies coding regions that are candidates for the gene mutated in the condition of interest. Finally, these candidates are

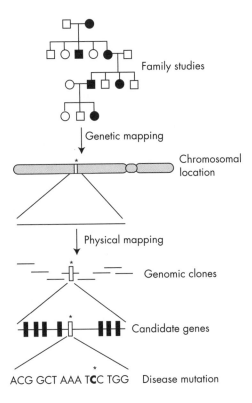

Family studies

Genetic mapping

Chromosomal location

Physical mapping

Genomic clones

Candidate genes

ACG GCT AAA TCC TGG   Disease mutation

Figure 2.2   From disease inheritance to mutant gene. A generalised scheme of the stages of disease gene identification is shown. Genetic mapping studies of informative pedigrees are used to define a minimal chromosomal fragment that confers the disease phenotype. Physical mapping studies of this region are then employed to assemble a series of genomic clones, within which candidate genes are identified. Further screening of candidate genes determines which gene bears mutations common to affected individuals but absent from those unaffected by the disease.

analysed to identify mutations that are common to individuals that present with the disease.

To these ends, a variety of key technologies and panels of mapping reagents have been developed. As necessitated by the nature of the problem, these methods range from cytogenetic studies of whole chromosomes or chromosome fragments to identification of single nucleotide changes in a specific disease gene.

Cytogenetic analysis

Although normally not visible by conventional microscopy, during mitosis replicated chromosomes condense as paired structures and align to a spindle to ensure accurate distribution of chromosomes to each daughter cell.

Experimentally, these condensed chromosomes can be stained and visualised by conventional light microscopy. Such preparations allow each chromosome pair to be unequivocally identified according to size and staining patterns. Together, this collection of stained chromosomes is termed a karyotype. Visual inspection of karyotypes is a fundamental tool used to identify abnormal chromosomes and is routinely applied in screens for some inherited diseases. For example, many Down's syndrome individuals are characterised by the presence of an extra copy of all, or part, of chromosome 21 that can be detected by biopsy and culture of fetal cells followed by chromosomal preparation and karyotyping. For other inherited conditions, cytogenetic defects are rare but can be highly informative in defining chromosomal regions of interest and have contributed to disease gene identification in several cases, including retinoblastoma, neurofibromatosis and Wilms' tumour.

Radiation hybrid cell lines provide a powerful sophistication to gene mapping. These cell cultures are generated by experimentally induced fusion *in vitro* of X-irradiated human cells with normal diploid cells of a distinct species, say mouse or hamster. Initially, the chromosomal constitution of the resulting hybrid cells is highly unstable. However, with subsequent cycles of replication and cell division a series of stable cell lines arises, each of which bears a specific human chromosome fragment (say 10 Mb in size) retained within a complement of the host species genome. The human chromosome regions specific for each line can be identified by screening with a selection of known chromosomal markers. This route has enabled assembly of panels of somatic cell hybrids that cover the entire human genome and which are of great value in large-scale gene mapping efforts and validation of candidate disease genes.

Detection of markers in such panels can be carried out by Southern blot hybridisation with specific DNA probes (Chapter 1). However, fluorescence *in situ* hybridisation (FISH) provides more detailed analysis of chromosomal rearrangements and chromosomal assignment of DNA markers in karyotypes of normal and radiation hybrid cells. In this assay, a cloned DNA molecule is labelled with a fluorescent marker and hybridised with a chromosomal preparation. The location of the hybridised fluorescent marker is then visualised in relation to the karyo-type morphology. Through use of chromosome-specific marker DNA molecules, each labelled with a distinct fluor, it is possible to assign whole chromosomes or chromosomal subregions (see Lichter, 1997, for review).

Genetic linkage maps

Any criterion can be used to study genetic linkage, provided there is a means of distinguishing the maternal and paternal alleles at each chromosomal locus. Historically, linkage markers have included differences in enzymatic activity and protein migration, but direct assay of nucleotide sequence differences now provides the most widely used and informative type of linkage marker. Naturally occurring DNA sequence polymorphisms occur irrespective of coding or non-coding regions of the genome and provide an essentially unlimited supply of genetic markers. A major goal of the Human Genome Project is to generate detailed linkage maps using markers that cover all regions of the genome. As discussed later, this is particularly important for mapping complex disease genes. Informative DNA markers can take a variety of forms.

Restriction fragment length polymorphisms (RFLPs) provide a common form of allelic marker for gene mapping. The principles underlying this method of analysis are shown in Figure 2.3. DNA restriction enzymes recognise and cleave DNA at specific nucleotide sequences (Chapter 1). In most cases, the restriction digest fragments generated from each allele at a given locus will be identical in size. Thus, a gene-specific radiolabelled probe would identify a single hybridising DNA fragment by Southern blot analysis for each of the two gene copies present in an individual. However, in some instances, variation in nucleotide sequence between maternal and paternal alleles results in loss of a restriction site at one of the two alleles. Hence, two hybridising bands are now apparent, allowing maternal and paternal alleles to be distinguished. Large numbers of such RFLPs have been identified using both anonymous DNA markers as well as markers of known genes.

Short tandem repeat polymorphisms (STRPs) are small repetitive nucleotide sequences that exist in tandem arrays of varying repeat numbers. Moreover, these tandem repeat DNA markers are of value for genome-wide searches since they are both abundant and dispersed throughout the genome. Dinucleotide CA repeats are most common, but trinucleotide and tetranucleotide repeats are also informative. Importantly, PCR-based approaches for STRP mapping have been developed.

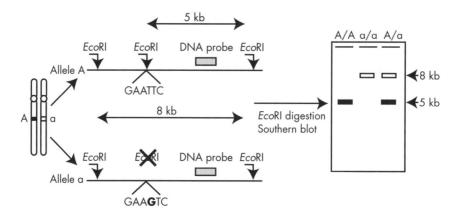

Figure 2.3 Restriction fragment length polymorphisms. DNA polymorphisms provide the major means of discriminating allelic markers. The principles underlying RFLPs are shown. The restriction enzyme *Eco*RI cuts genomic DNA specifically at the nucleotide sequence GAATTC. At a given genetic locus, variation of a single nucleotide is sufficient to create or destroy an *Eco*RI restriction site to generate two distinct alleles (A or a). Southern blot analysis using a DNA probe specific for this locus is sufficient to distinguish individuals that bear two copies of the A allele or two copies of the a allele or are heterozygous (A/a) at this locus.

This not only facilitates rapid analyses, but also enables marker information to be stored as data files in the form of oligonucleotide primer sequences, rather than as cloned DNA fragments.

As part of the Human Genome Project, a collaborative effort of several groups has applied combinations of RFLPs, STRPs, anonymous gene markers and known genes to generate a saturated human genetic linkage map of over 5000 loci with a mean resolution of 0.7 cM (Murray *et al.*, 1994). This resource promises to be of great value in facilitating mapping of disease susceptibility genes.

Physical linkage maps

By measuring genetic linkage between disease phenotype and known DNA markers, a small chromosomal fragment can be defined within which is the disease gene of interest. Further progress requires physical mapping, with the challenge being to clone the relevant chromosomal region and identify candidate genes that may be mutated in the disease.

In this respect, it should be borne in mind that the resolution afforded by genetic mapping is generally much less than that of physical maps. Genetic linkage maps measure the frequency of recombination between loci, whereas physical maps measure the distance in nucleotides between genes on a chromosome. An approximate relationship is that 1 cM is equivalent to 1000 kb at the nucleotide level. Thus, two loci considered to be close at 3 cM distance in a genetic linkage map approximate to 3000 kb on a physical map. As a typical gene might cover 100 kb, the chromosomal fragment defined by genetic linkage could contain 30 or more genes, of which only one is mutated in the disease under investigation.

Yeast artificial chromosome (YAC) libraries of human genomic DNA provide the necessary intermediate between chromosomal fragments, defined by genetic analysis, and cloned DNA. Each YAC clone within the library contains a distinct, and relatively large, genomic DNA fragment (200–400 kb) that is maintained in yeast as an autonomously replicating DNA molecule in addition to the normal yeast genome.

Importantly, there is redundancy of clones within the library in that the fragment present in each clone is designed to include regions common to others. In this way, overlapping YAC clones can be assembled in contiguous arrays (contigs) that reconstitute the order of DNA fragments in the chromosome. Thus, large chromosomal fragments can be represented as a series of overlapping YAC clones, creating a physical map.

A further feature of the co-ordinated utilisation of YAC libraries for disease gene mapping is the integration of physical maps with cytogenetic and linkage maps. STRPs identified in YAC clones can be used to map chromosomal fragments by FISH (see above), so allowing YAC contigs to be ordered on chromosomes. Sequence-tagged-sites (STSs) constitute marker probes that are also useful in this respect. An STS is any small (200–500 bp) sequence that is unique within the genome and can be anonymous DNA or represent part of a gene. Linkage of STSs can be established by screening combinations on radiation hybrid panels and YACs, their presence or absence being readily tested by PCR. In this way, chromosomal rearrangements, which are often of great value in defining the limits of a disease locus, can be mapped relative to genetic markers. In a recent effort, an STS map of 15 000 distinct loci was developed by these routes. In turn, this framework map was used to map 16 000 gene-based STSs (Schuler *et al.*, 1996). Such a detailed human gene map provides an important resource, linking genetic and physical maps with nucleotide databases, that will enable disease gene identification once a small genomic region has been defined.

With the relevant genomic clones to hand, there remains the

problem of identifying the specific disease gene within this region. A variety of methods are available that screen for the presence of characteristic motifs of genes, including conservation of sequences between human and other species. Validation of candidate coding regions can then be carried out by other methods such as screening for expression in tissues affected in the disease state and direct DNA sequence determination to identify mutations common to affected individuals but absent in those who do not carry the disease gene. In some cases, such as fibroblast growth factor receptor 3 in achondroplasia, RET receptor tyrosine kinase in multiple endocrine neoplasia and Hirshsprung's disease, pre-existing knowledge of candidate gene function in relation to disease pathophysiology has been invaluable in discriminating between candidate coding regions.

Complex disease traits

In contrast to single-gene defects subject to simple Mendelian inheritance, identification of gene mutations that contribute to polygenic or multifactorial conditions present much greater technical challenges. Complex disease traits result from allelic mutations of several interacting loci. Such mutations tend to be relatively weak alleles, each of which is not sufficient in itself to induce disease but which can act in an additive or multiplicative manner to confer susceptibility to disease, often in conjunction with environmental factors. The contributions of multiple genetic components, as well as non-genetic factors, result in non-Mendelian patterns of inheritance for such susceptibility genes. As a consequence, polygenic traits are more prevalent but require distinct methods of genetic analysis. The challenge for disease gene identification in complex traits lies in seeking to define multiple interacting weak mutant alleles in the absence of any biological markers or knowledge of the mode of inheritance.

Assessing genetic contribution to complex diseases

A genetic contribution to complex disease traits is generally established by estimating an individual's risk of disease occurrence within affected families, and makes extensive use of twins and adoption cases that include affected individuals. These reveal that, if there is already an affected family member, the risk of an individual developing the condition increases multiplicatively. Thus, in schizophrenia, individuals with an affected sibling were found to have a 9% risk, compared with a 1% lifetime risk in the general population. This risk increases to 16% if both an affected sibling and parent are known within the family. Similarly, although non-identical twins have increased risks similar to that of normal siblings, monozygotic twins (who in principle have identical genes) have a 46–48% lifetime risk of schizophrenia (Karayiorgou and Gogos, 1997). In Alzheimer's disease, family studies are complicated by late onset of the condition, but sibling risk is estimated at 3–14%, whereas among monozygotic twins between 40% and 50% concordance has been observed. A strong genetic effect has also been observed in autism, for which sibling risk is 2.9%, but concordance among monozygotic twins can be as high as 60%. In contrast, concordance among dizygotic twins is very low, indicating that several loci are likely to be involved as well as environmental factors. Clearly, in such cases a genetic component is apparent, but inheritance is not Mendelian.

Mapping complex disease susceptibility genes

As with single-gene defects, the aim is to use genetic mapping to locate susceptibility loci to small chromosomal fragments that are amenable to subsequent physical mapping. However, the sample size required for linkage analysis increases as the genetic effect of the mutation decreases. Together with epidemiological factors, such as late age of disease onset, this restricts the resolution of genetic studies to broad regions of interest, no smaller than 2–5 cM for small-effect genes.

Tests for linkage in complex diseases require approaches that not only make no assumptions about the mode of inheritance, but also provide sufficient statistical power to detect weak alleles. In such cases, linkage studies apply genome-wide searches using highly polymorphic genetic markers, together with specific statistical programs. Rather than measure recombination, affected-sibling pair analysis determines whether two affected siblings within a pedigree family share more marker alleles identical by descent (IBD) than expected by chance. A complementary route of analysis is the affected pedigree member (APM) method. This approach seeks correlation of marker associations common to affected members of several distinct pedigrees, rather than looking within a family pedigree. APM has the advantage that there is no requirement for rare families with multiple affected individuals and thus it is suited to analysis of late-onset diseases, such as Alzheimer's.

However, there is a requirement that candidate markers are first identified and so it is useful for further testing of candidate regions identified initially through linkage analysis.

Detailed gene maps resulting from the Human Genome Project will be vital to improving mapping of susceptibility genes for such complex traits. For some conditions, correlation with Mendelian conditions that map to the same candidate genomic regions and share similar phenotypic properties provides supporting information. For example, Marfan syndrome (15q21.1) co-segregates with schizophrenia. The Marfan syndrome gene has recently been cloned as fibrillin 1, facilitating molecular analysis of the involvement of this gene in schizophrenia. Similarly, a region of chromosome 22 implicated in schizophrenia overlaps with a region implicated in velocardiofacial syndrome (VCFS). Consistent with a schizophrenia susceptibility locus in this region of overlap, 29% of VCFS patients also develop schizophrenia.

Future prospects

Gene mapping technology has progressed to a stage where identification of causal mutations in single-gene defects is now fairly routine and analysis of complex disease traits can be approached (Schafer and Hawkins, 1998). The Human Genome Project has already provided nucleotide sequence information on approximately 50% of all human genes, and completion of this database can be expected in the near future. With the related improvements in the quality of genetic and physical linkage maps, we can anticipate greatly improved efficiency of disease gene-cloning efforts that will come to focus increasingly on analysis of known candidate genes.

The availability of a cloned disease gene is of immediate value in terms of screening for the presence or absence of mutations that confer predisposition to the condition. In multifactorial disease, the presence of susceptibility alleles related to an individual's response to certain foreign compounds could prove to be extremely valuable in preventative efforts to minimise disease risk. Gene mapping technology can also be applied to the identification of genetic components that contribute to phenotypic phenomena, other than disease, that are observed to vary within human populations. For example, variations observed between individual patient responses to specific drug regimens are thought to reflect differential action of drug-metabolising enzymes that may result from specific combinations of susceptibility loci. The identification of such loci (pharmacogenomics) would facilitate development of screening procedures that could contribute towards optimising specific drug regimens for individual patients.

As a result of these and other applications, a greatly increased demand for DNA sequence information can be expected in the near future. For a given gene, deletions, rearrangements, or specific nucleotide changes that occur at high frequency are relatively easy to detect. However, in some cases, such as breast cancer susceptibility genes *BRCA1* and *BRCA2*, it is becoming apparent that mutations are scattered throughout the large coding regions of these genes (Kahn, 1996). Here, routine high-throughput screening across the entire coding region is a much more demanding task. Moreover, it should be noted that mutations affecting gene transcription will not be identified by this route and require additional knowledge of the gene regulatory elements, or development of RNA screening or antigen screening technologies.

At the heart of efforts to improve methods of high-throughput DNA sequencing for diagnostic purposes are high-density oligonucleotide arrays (Marshall and Hodgson, 1998). Development of such arrays combines the principles and specificity of nucleic acid hybridisation with the existing manufacturing base of silicon chip production, resulting in the creation of so-called DNA chips. New nucleic acid synthesis technologies now allow as many as 400 000 distinct oligonucleotide sequences to be immobilised in an ordered array on a chip 1.6 cm^2. These immobilised oligonucleotide arrays are then used to probe an unknown set of nucleic acid sequences, utilising the specificity of complementary nucleic acid hybridisation. The nucleic acid populations to be screened can be labelled, say with a fluorescent marker, and DNA hybridised to specific oligonucleotides is then detected by scanning the high-density array with a modified confocal microscope. By careful monitoring of hybridisation conditions, only 100% sequence identity is revealed by hybridisation, allowing single base changes to be identified. In principle, arrays of this density would enable all 50 000 genes currently identified to be screened on only four chips.

For specific disease genes, polymorphisms and single nucleotide changes could be identified, and applications in analysis of complex genetic traits, identification of pathogens and forensic analysis can also be envisaged. Within the pharmaceutical industry DNA chip technology could also be applied in high-throughput screening of compounds for induced changes in gene expression profiles. However, although the power and specificity of this approach have been proved in principle, major challenges remain in developing this technology for routine diagnostic applications, including improvements in automation, miniaturisation, sample handling and data management. Most importantly in terms of patient care, the effectiveness of such assays in accurate diagnosis must be demonstrated.

Continued application and development of the technologies described here offer the prospect of a wealth of information relating to both the current and prospective health status of an individual. This will be of considerable value in disease diagnosis, preventative medicine and the development of more specialised screening programmes and individual drug regimens. However, assimilation of such information on an individual and their relatives is highly sensitive, and also presents potential psychological, social and economic implications. Such consequences need to be considered with great care.

References

Kahn P (1996) Coming to grips with genes and risk. *Science* 274: 496–498.

Karayiorgou M, Gogos J A (1997) A turning point in schizophrenia genetics. *Neuron* 19: 967–979.

Lichter P (1997) Multicolor FISHing: what's the catch? *Trends Genet* 13: 475–479.

Marshall A, Hodgson J (1998) DNA chips: an array of possibilities. *Nature Biotechnol* 16: 27–31.

Murray J C, Buetwow K H, Weber J L, *et al.* (1994) A comprehensive human linkage map with centimorgan density. Cooperative Human Linkage Center (CHLC). *Science* 265: 2049–2054.

Schafer A J, Hawkins J R (1998) DNA variation and the future of human genetics. *Nature Biotechnol* 16: 33–44

Schuler G D, Boguski M S, Steware E A, *et al.* (1996) A gene map of the human genome. *Science* 274: 540–546.

Further reading

Lander E S (1996) The new genomics: global views of biology. *Science* 274: 536–539.

3

Gene cloning

Nicola Hardwick and Richard G Vile

In the early 1970s, techniques were developed that enabled the cutting and joining of DNA molecules, and as a result manipulation of genetic material became possible. The exact mechanism by which exogenous DNA can be taken up by cells has not been fully elucidated, but what is known is that if a piece of DNA is not integrated into the host DNA it will be lost during subsequent cell division (Watt *et al.*, 1992). For the introduced DNA to be replicated as the cell replicates, it must contain a replicon (origin of replication/ori). The standard method, therefore, is to attach the DNA in question to a suitable replicon known as a 'vector'.

The most commonly used vectors are small plasmids and bacteriophages. Successful insertion of foreign DNA results in the construction of 'chimaeric DNA'. It is the construction of such chimaeras that is the basis of recombinant DNA technology. This process has been termed 'gene cloning' (Figure 3.1) because a line of genetically identical organisms (all containing the same DNA construct) can be propagated and grown in bulk, hence amplifying the DNA construct (Watt *et al.*, 1992).

How this is done can be summarised as follows:

1   Foreign DNA must be characterised, isolated and purified from its source.
2   Vector DNA must be isolated, purified and cut with restriction enzymes in such a way as to allow insertion of the foreign DNA fragment.
3   The DNA must then be joined and closed.
4   The ligated DNA is then introduced into a host cell, which allows its propagation *in vitro*.
5   The effectiveness of the DNA splicing is examined and successful recombinants selected.

Although elegantly simple in concept, the process of gene cloning is technically quite demanding.

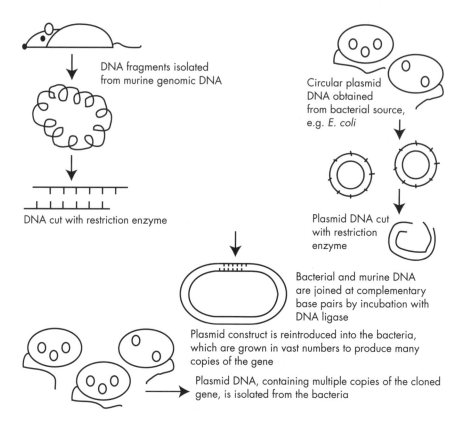

DNA fragments isolated from murine genomic DNA

Circular plasmid DNA obtained from bacterial source, e.g. *E. coli*

DNA cut with restriction enzyme

Plasmid DNA cut with restriction enzyme

Bacterial and murine DNA are joined at complementary base pairs by incubation with DNA ligase

Plasmid construct is reintroduced into the bacteria, which are grown in vast numbers to produce many copies of the gene

Plasmid DNA, containing multiple copies of the cloned gene, is isolated from the bacteria

Figure 3.1 The process of gene cloning.

Plasmids

Plasmids are small circular extrachromosomal DNA elements found in bacteria which possess their own origin of replication and so are able to replicate independently in bacteria. Their natural function is the exchange of genes between bacteria such as genes for antibiotic resistance (Maniatis *et al.*, 1982).

Use of plasmids in cloning

Plasmids (Figure 3.2) are used as 'cloning vectors' in that, once they have been isolated from bacteria, the gene to be cloned is inserted and the resulting construct reintroduced into bacteria. The bacteria can then be grown in large numbers (allowing the plasmid to replicate many times) and the DNA subsequently obtained by conventional means (see page 38).

Plasmids are not generally used in the form in which they are found in nature; commercially available plasmids have been customised in some of the following ways:

1   Adding sequences which are recognised by certain restriction enzymes, thereby permitting manipulation of the plasmid. Often a 'polylinker' sequence is included, which contains several concurrent enzyme sites, so allowing a variety of cloning strategies.

2   Removal of non-essential DNA to make the plasmid smaller and thus easier to handle *in vitro* (this may include the removal of unwanted restriction sites).

3   Insertion of genes that allow easy selection/screening of recombinants, e.g. *lacZ*, ampicillin resistance (see below).

4   Replacing the natural ori with a mutant ori that allows 'relaxed copy number control', i.e. the plasmid continues to replicate after the bacterium has stopped growing. In a natural situation such a property would perhaps not be of benefit to the symbiotic plasmid or the bacterium, but in molecular biology it is a useful way of obtaining a higher yield of DNA (Brady *et al.*, 1995).

Circular, independently replicating, extrachromosomal DNA also occurs naturally in yeast and mammalian cells but is less suitable for gene cloning.

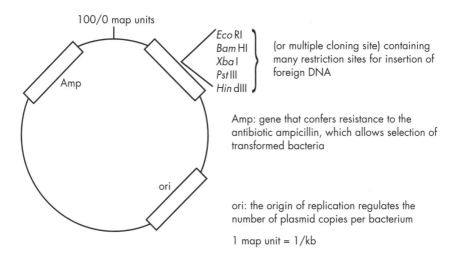

Figure 3.2   Essential features of a plasmid.

How plasmids are used

Initially, the plasmid DNA is digested (cut) with a restriction endo-nuclease. These are enzymes that cut double-stranded DNA at specific sites that they recognise in the DNA sequence (Maniatis *et al.*, 1982). They are obtained from a variety of bacteria, in which their natural function is to act as a defence against foreign DNA, particularly bacteriophages (Brady *et al.*, 1995). Bacteria protect their own DNA from digestion by their own restriction enzymes by methylation, which blocks many restriction enzymes. If bacteriophage DNA is cut by a bacterial enzyme, it cannot infect that strain of bacteria, although it may be able to infect another strain with different restriction en-zymes. Mammalian DNA can usually be cut *in vitro* with restriction enzymes despite often being methylated. This is because methylation in eukaryotic cells has a different function from that in prokaryotic cells (bacteria) and does not protect the DNA from restriction en-zymes.

A suitable restriction site on the plasmid is used to cut it open to allow the insertion of the insert DNA. Most restriction enzymes yield protruding cohesive 5′ termini (so-called 'sticky ends'; Figure 3.3) which can be joined by complementary base pairing to other DNA mol-ecules.

Six-base cutters are commonly used because they tend to cut DNA into fragments that are small enough to handle. Blunt-end ligation has the disadvantage of generating a DNA fragment that is able to rejoin without the insert (self-ligation). Also, sticky-ended fragments that have been cut with a single enzyme can self-ligate by base pairing, although such self-ligation can be reduced by dephosphorylation of the vector DNA.

A sticky-ended vector with different ends cannot in theory self-ligate because the overhanging ends are not compatible and so will not anneal. Sticky-end ligation with different ends has the added advantage of allowing 'directional cloning' since the insert should only be able to be inserted into the vector in one direction. Obviously, this requires that the correct ends be generated on the insert DNA prior to ligation (this can be achieved by the use of shuttle vectors or PCR technology) (Brady *et al.*, 1994).

If 'same end' ligation is used, subsequent analysis will be required to check whether the insert has been cloned into the vector in the correct orientation (Figure 3.4).

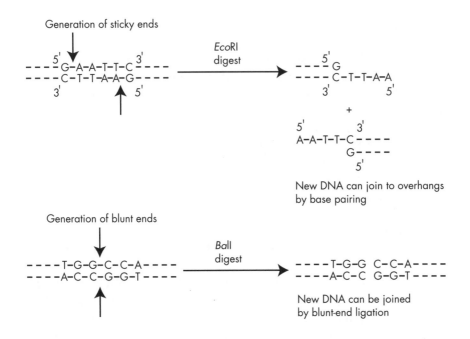

Figure 3.3 Cutting with restriction enzymes.

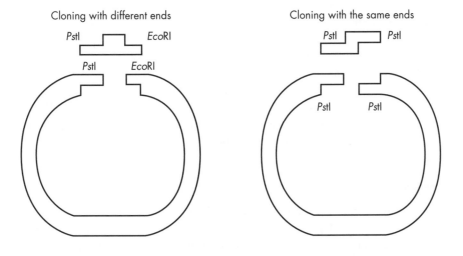

Figure 3.4 Different cloning strategies.

DNA ligases

The enzyme DNA ligase acts on the two ends of DNA generated by digestion and reconnects the phosphate backbone. Sticky-end ligations tend to be far more efficient because the compatible ends have a natural, albeit weak, affinity for each other. However, blunt-end ligation can be useful since, in theory, it allows the joining of any two DNA fragments without the need for compatible ends.

Transformation

Following ligation, the products of a ligation reaction are introduced back into host cells, usually bacteria such as *Escherichia coli*, so that the plasmid construct can be amplified.

Bacterial cells are said to be 'transformed' when DNA is introduced, whereas mammalian cells are said to be 'transfected' (Brady *et al.*, 1994). Bacteria will spontaneously take in extraneous DNA although the process is of very low efficiency. Therefore, 'competent bacteria' are commonly used, so-called because they have been specially treated in order to make them more amenable to DNA uptake.

Selection/screening

Once the bacteria have been incubated with the ligation products under suitable conditions, they are allowed to grow on selective media. Owing to the low efficiency of transformation, it is necessary to separate the non-transformed cells from those which have taken up the DNA (Brady *et al.*, 1995). These positive bacterial clones are said to be either 'selected' or 'screened' depending upon the method used.

Selection (Figure 3.5)

The bacteria are transformed with a plasmid that contains a 'selectable marker' such as a gene encoding antibiotic resistance (e.g. ampicillin resistance). The cells are then plated onto media containing the antibiotic in question. The few cells which have taken up the plasmid will express the antibiotic resistance gene and will be able to grow on the media, while the untransformed cells will be killed by the antibiotic (Brady *et al.*, 1995).

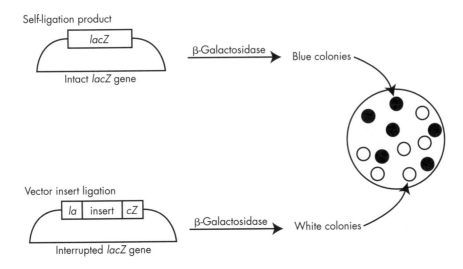

Self-ligation product

lacZ

Intact *lacZ* gene

β-Galactosidase → Blue colonies

Vector insert ligation

la | insert | cZ

Interrupted *lacZ* gene

β-Galactosidase → White colonies

Figure 3.5   Selection of transformed bacteria.

Screening

An example of this is when the plasmid contains a gene for an enzyme, the activity of which can be easily detected with chromogenic substrates that either remain soluble or precipitate in solution. A common example of this is plasmids containing a gene called *lacZ*, which allows the conversion of a colourless compound called X-gal to a blue precipitate. The plasmid is constructed such that the *lacZ* gene spans the cloning site in the vector. Thus, if a gene is successfully inserted into the vector, the *lacZ* gene is interrupted and function is lost. Any bacteria transformed with such a construct will not be able to metabolise the X-gal substrate and will not produce any blue product. A plasmid which has self-ligated, and therefore has an intact *lacZ* gene, will be able to convert X-gal to its blue product and will therefore be distinguishable from the former. Such screening methods are often used in conjunction with selection methods.

Purification and further analysis of plasmid DNA

At this point, the common way to proceed is to pick a number of the selected/screened bacterial clones from the plate and transfer them to small aliquots of liquid media containing the selective agent. These individual cultures are encouraged to grow, and DNA is subsequently obtained from them. Such preparations of DNA are often termed 'minipreps' since they yield small amounts of DNA for further analysis.

Purification of plasmid DNA from bacterial DNA is possible because of the circular nature of plasmid DNA. The bacterial cell contents are exposed to denaturing conditions, which cause the DNA strands to come apart. Once returned to renaturing conditions, the complex bacterial chromosomal DNA is unable to realign with its matching strands. In contrast, the strands of circular plasmid DNA remain linked and so are able to reanneal efficiently. The intact plasmid can then be easily removed from the denatured bacterial chromosomal DNA (Brady *et al.*, 1995).

The resulting DNA can then be analysed to determine if the gene has been correctly cloned into the vector, with two methods being commonly used:

1   *Restriction enzyme analysis.* In the same way that restriction enzymes are used to generate the required components for ligation, they can also be used to check whether a particular ligation has been successful.
2   *PCR analysis* (see Chapter 5 for details). This is performed using primers which anneal to certain areas of the vector in such a way that a positive PCR band will only be generated if the required construct has been made.

Finally, once the correct construct has been identified, the bacterial culture from which it was isolated can be grown up in bulk and a larger amount of DNA (usually termed a maxiprep) can be made.

Recombinant DNA technology – use of DNA chimaeras

Once a pure, concentrated preparation of the construct DNA has been obtained, it can be used to introduce the gene into the target cells, in which, it is hoped, it will be expressed. Numerous transfection techniques have been developed to increase the efficiency of DNA uptake including (reviewed in Kriegler, 1990):

1   calcium phosphate precipitation
2   DEAE–dextran
3   cationic liposomes
4   biolistics/gene guns
5   electroporation.

Despite the use of these techniques, however, a good transfection rate of mammalian cells results in only approximately 10% of the cells receiving DNA, with less than 1% of these cells being able to form stable transfectants.

When using vectors that integrate into the host cell genome, it should be possible to generate a stable transfectant, as the gene will be passed on each time the cell divides. Such cellular clones must be selected from the mass of untransduced cells in the same way that transformed bacteria are selected from non-transformed cells. Again this is commonly done using antibiotic resistance genes contained in the plasmid.

Cells that have taken up and expressed the plasmid will be able to grow in media containing the antibiotic in question (obviously an antibiotic that is usually toxic to mammalian cells). This small number of cells can be selected in culture from the majority of non-transfected cells, which will die when cultured with the antibiotic.

The surviving cells will obviously then divide and produce daughter cells. If the construct has been integrated, it will be replicated along with the cellular DNA at mitosis, so any daughter cells will also contain the same construct. Therefore, a line of genetically identical cells (clones) containing the new DNA will be generated. Different clones can then be examined for expression of the required gene (Watt *et al.*, 1992).

Uses of gene cloning

The cloning of genes and their subsequent introduction into cells *in vitro* has been of considerable use in classical genetics, in that it has allowed greater analysis of gene structure and function. However, it has also had a significant effect on healthcare, and promises much more for the future. Some of these potential uses are described below.

Recombinant proteins

Where gene cloning has had perhaps the greatest impact on healthcare is in the production of recombinant proteins. Once the gene for a therapeutic protein has been cloned, it is inserted into an expression vector, where it is placed under the control of a strong promoter (Chapter 1). The type of promoter used will depend on whether the protein is to be made in bacterial, yeast or mammalian cells. Such a construct can then be introduced into a host cell, where large-scale production of the protein occurs.

Table 3.1 Examples of recombinant proteins in clinical use

Protein	Therapeutic use	Year introduced
Human insulin	Diabetes mellitus	1982
Human growth hormone	Growth hormone deficiency in children	1985
Tissue-type plasminogen activator	Myocardial infarction	1987
Erythropoietin	Anaemia due to chronic renal failure	1989
Granulocyte colony-stimulating factor (G-CSF)	Neutropenia following chemotherapy	1991
Granulocyte–macrophage colony-stimulating factor (GM-CSF)	Myeloid reconstitution after bone marrow transplantation	1991
Factor VIII	Haemophilia A	1992
Interferon-α	Chronic hepatitis A and C	1992
IL-2	Immunotherapy of malignant disease	1993

This has enabled pure human proteins to be mass produced for the treatment of disease. Although, strictly speaking, it is the DNA that is 'recombinant', the proteins produced by cloning are usually referred to as 'recombinant', even when they are identical to naturally occurring proteins (Brady *et al.*, 1995).

The first recombinant human protein to be used clinically was insulin in 1982, followed by many others such as growth hormone, erythropoietin and factor VIII for haemophilia (Table 3.1).

Prior to recombinant DNA technology, the usual source of these proteins was animal or human tissue. Such purification was not only time-consuming, but carried considerable risks to the patient regarding the transmission of infection (such as HIV in contaminated human factor VIII and Creutzfeldt–Jakob disease in bovine growth hormone). In addition, proteins purified from an animal source can often be recognised as foreign by the immune system.

Genetic disease

Once a gene has been fully characterised and cloned, pathological abnormalities in the gene can be more easily investigated at the DNA, RNA and protein levels. This can lead to a greater understanding of the disease process and allow the development of methods to screen patient DNA for mutated genes. Unfortunately, however, many genetic diseases are as yet untreatable (e.g. Huntington's chorea), and assistance may be limited to genetic counselling.

Gene therapy

The treatment of genetic disorders (including cancer) by correcting the underlying abnormality through gene therapy is now becoming an achievable goal (see Chapter 6). However, before gene therapy for any genetic disorder can be developed, there is one fundamental requirement, namely that the therapeutic gene be cloned and sequenced so that it is fully characterised and readily available in bulk in the required form. This is always the first step in the development of a gene therapy approach and is necessary before the problems of gene delivery, targeting and expression can be addressed.

Cancer therapy

As well as recombinant cytokines (see Chapter 10) and the promise of gene therapy (see Chapter 6), gene cloning offers another possibility in malignant disease, namely tumour-specific peptides. Mutated oncoproteins can, in some cases, generate cytotoxic T-lymphocyte (CTL) responses; therefore, peptide fragments of such proteins could be used to 'immunise' patients against their own tumours. Genes encoding tumour antigens that are recognised by CD8+ T cells can be cloned and then further analysed for suitable epitopes (Boon et al., 1992).

B-cell lymphoma is a good example of a tumour that could be treated in this way. This tumour arises from the clonal proliferation of a single B cell. Thus, each B-cell lymphoma produces a distinct antibody with a unique V region (binding site). Recombinant DNA technology has made it possible to clone the V region from lymphoma cells and construct a recombinant vaccine by fusing the V-region protein with other proteins such as GM-CSF to make it more immunogenic (Brady et al., 1995).

An alternative to using tumour antigens in peptide form is to immunise the patient with the recombinant DNA. Such 'DNA vaccination' relies on the principle that suitable tissue such as muscle tissue is transfected with the DNA, and hence that the peptide is produced *in vivo*, with the generation of a CTL response to the tumour epitope (Robinson and

Torres, 1997). This approach can also be applied to infectious disease (see below), allergy and autoimmunity (Robinson and Torres, 1997).

Vaccines for infectious diseases

The cloning and expression of genes from infectious organisms allows the production of recombinant proteins that may be used as vaccines against the organism in question (Brady *et al.*, 1995). Unfortunately, this approach has been hindered by the inability to generate proteins in a soluble but immunogenic form. However, one recombinant vaccine that has been produced is the vaccine against hepatitis B virus. This has been developed by cloning the surface protein of the virus and expressing it in yeast cells, which then produce particles that closely resemble the natural viral protein. When used as a vaccine, a strong immune response is seen against hepatitis B virus in immunised individuals (Brady *et al.*, 1995).

Recombinant antibodies

In their natural form, antibodies can induce death of viruses, mammalian cells and bacteria by 'antibody-directed cell-mediated cytotoxicity' or by complement-mediated lysis.

The genes which encode for antibodies can be cloned and modified, allowing the production of antibodies with reduced immunogenicity, greater affinity and in some cases new functions (Chester and Hawkins, 1995). These can then be used therapeutically in a variety of ways including:

1   carrying radionucleotides, enzymes, genes, drugs or toxins to target cells;
2   blocking binding of ligands (e.g. hormones with their receptors);
3   neutralising toxins.

Specific antibodies can be generated to most target antigens and, therefore, the clinical potential for antibody-based therapy is enormous. At present, clinical trials involving a wide range of diseases are under way, including cancer, transplant rejection, viral infection, autoimmunity, toxic shock, restenosis and haemolytic disease (Chester and Hawkins, 1995). Traditionally, antibodies have been produced from hybridomas or animals, but cloning and modification can produce recombinant antibodies of greater efficiency. Murine antibodies, for example, have a short half-life in humans because they are recognised as foreign. In the same way, cloned human proteins are not recognised by the patient's immune system; thus, cloned human antibodies do not invoke an immune response after repeated administration (Chester and Hawkins, 1995).

Usually it is the single-chain (Sc) Fv (which contains both heavy- and light-chain variable regions) that is used to develop antibody-based therapeutic molecules (McCafferty *et al.*, 1990). These Fv chains are readily cloned and expressed in bacteria, and can even be incorporated into fusion molecules. ScFvs can also be displayed as functional antibody fragments on the surface of bacteriophages, allowing the selection of potentially useful antibodies from vast libraries (McCafferty *et al.*, 1990).

Antibody-targeted cancer therapy

In some cases, the identification of a suitable 'tumour antigen' allows the production of corresponding recombinant antibodies which can be used to target tumour cells for the following purposes:

1   *Tumour imaging.* This has been achieved using monoclonal antibodies (see Chapter 11), but is often no more effective than standard methods. This is thought to be because only a low proportion of the antibody actually reaches the tumour (Chester and Hawkins, 1996).
2   *Tumour killing.* Many different effector molecules can be linked to antibodies to cause targeted killing, including cytotoxic drugs, immunotoxins, prodrugs and radionucleotides.

In the case of radiosensitive tumours, e.g. lymphoma, antibody-guided radiotherapy can result in prolonged remission (Press *et al.*, 1993). Newer methods using immunotoxins look promising, such as the induction of apoptosis in acute leukaemia using an antibody-targeted inhibitor of a tyrosine kinase (Uckun *et al.*, 1995). Antibodies have also been used in prodrug therapy (antibody-directed enzyme–prodrug therapy, ADEPT) to localise an enzyme to tumour sites. A non-toxic prodrug is then administered and is activated by the enzyme to produce a cytotoxic drug. The first ADEPT clinical trial was carried out in colorectal cancer patients using a benzoic acid mustard prodrug and showed encouraging results (Bagshawe *et al.*, 1995).

Gene therapy for cancer using antibody genes

It may in theory be possible to deliver genes encoding antibodies to patients' cells so that the therapeutic antibody is produced *in situ*. If such antibodies were directed at appropriate targets they then could be used to inhibit tumour growth (Deshane *et al.*, 1994). For example, tumours known to be dependent on growth factors or hormones could be transfected with genes encoding neutralising antibodies to the factor in question.

The wider implications of gene cloning

The ability to clone genes is now commonplace in molecular biology laboratories. Furthermore, it now is trivial to alter the sequences of cloned genes to introduce novel mutations which may affect the form or function of the encoded protein. In addition, non-coding sequences of DNA can also be cloned and manipulated in identical ways.

This sort of investigative power has opened almost limitless horizons in basic genetic research. Once a sequence of DNA is available, cloning and associated techniques mean that it can be studied, altered, understood and used to a degree that was previously impossible. However, the implications of the sheer power of the cloning technology reach far beyond the research laboratory bench, and the issues involved should be considered by all who work in this area. Thus, the advent of molecular cloning has already raised, and is likely to continue to raise, impassioned debate in social, ethical, legal, commercial and religious domains. Some of the aspects of these debates are raised below in order that all those workers in the field are at least aware of the passions and implications of the methodology that is now routinely used in thousands of laboratories across the world.

Arguments for and against gene cloning

Arguments for gene cloning

The ability to identify a gene that is involved in disease, and then to clone it, has opened up a genuine revolution in medicine in the areas of both treatment and diagnosis. There is now real hope that genetic therapies can be used to correct diseases in which genes have been mutated/lost (see Chapter 6). Thus, cloned versions of genes that are defective in diseases ranging from cystic fibrosis and Duchenne muscular dystrophy through to cancer and viral diseases can be used to correct the disease phenotypes in affected tissues and, by inference, in the whole patient. Moreover, gene cloning allows enormous benefits in the area of diagnosis of disease.

Cloning and sequencing of the genes from patients can provide diagnostic information that was previously not obtainable. Often, early, asymptomatic diagnosis can lead to early intervention and prophylactic treatment, which greatly increases the chances of treatment success. Such diagnoses can be made with exquisite precision at the level of the DNA sequence of genes known to be affected in the disease.

Gene cloning also offers the potential to produce therapeutic proteins at levels that would vastly reduce the cost associated with protein purification and/or chemical synthesis from pre-existing sources. Industrial-scale production of these proteins, such as human insulin to treat diabetes or clotting factors to treat haemophilia, expressed from cloned genes in the appropriate vehicles (such as bacterial expression systems), may soon help patients who previously had very limited or no therapeutic options. The nature of the 'appropriate vehicle' is, of itself, a controversial topic. Thus, it is now readily possible to engineer various animal species to express human genes, for example in their milk, allowing easy, large-scale purification of the therapeutic protein (see Chapter 8). However, using bacterial expression systems to produce proteins in higher animal species such as goats, sheep and cows has already raised ferocious objections from various quarters, including animal rights groups (see below).

Cloning also promises to have a dramatic effect in commercial spheres in which the expression of certain types of genes can offer improvements over existing products. Already, there are fruits and vegetables on sale in which genes have been inserted to improve the field life (preventing rotting or attack by parasites), shelf life (slowing ripening) or taste (Chapter 8). In theory, this use of gene cloning seems attractive in its ability to improve the quality and cost-effectiveness of commercial products. However, it is often argued that it is rash to sell such modified foodstuffs in the absence of clear knowledge of how the inserted genes will affect the consumer and the environment.

Arguments against gene cloning

Very few people would argue that the huge potential benefits to medical science afforded by the ability to clone genes of different types do not justify the development of this technology. However, the rapid progression of cloning abilities also raises very legitimate concerns that must be addressed to ensure that gene cloning does not have disastrous consequences.

Several groups suggest that any tinkering with the very substance of life itself, i.e. DNA, is inappropriate and is best left to divine forces. However, some very dedicated religious scientists would argue the converse – the ability to modify diseased genes in the interests of medical science is one of the ultimate justifications for science itself. Whatever the religious arguments, there are also a host of social, ethical and commercial issues raised by cloning which must be appreciated.

For instance, just as the potential benefits to medical science of cloning disease-associated genes are huge from a diagnostic/treatment point of view, so the social implications could be catastrophic to the very set of patients whom the technology seeks to benefit. Thus, insurance companies have rapidly appreciated the value of the technology to exclude apparently healthy patients from cover if genetic tests are available to predict any diseases that they may develop in years to come. These decisions can affect the awards of medical or life insurance policies as well as mortgages and even job offers.

In addition, the ability to map and clone genes associated with behavioural patterns, rather than with medical conditions, also threatens to create social upheaval. Already there are reports of linkage of genes with traits such as homosexuality, dyslexia and even intelligence. The identification of such genes will inevitably lead to the stigmatisation of social and ethnic groups if they are found to express, or be deficient in, some of these 'behavioural' genes and could be used by different factions to justify prejudicial victimisation and suppression. It is but a short step from these arguments to the instigation of eugenic regimes based in large part on the ability to clone different sets of genes associated with social, ethnic or behavioural traits.

This raises the ever-present concern that gene cloning will eventually provide a weapon much more powerful than either the gun or prejudice in the ambitions of men to create the eugenically pure master race and to eliminate other traits considered at any particular time or place to be undesirable. In its most benign form, this concern is expressed through the possible wish of parents to 'compose' their children of the most desirable traits through the use of cloned genes inserted into the sperm, eggs or fetus. Currently, such notions are dismissed as impossible, as the genes required to produce, for example, 'intelligence' or 'good looks' are not only unidentified (partly because the concepts themselves are unidentifiable on a global scale) but also undeliverable. However, the concerns that such social engineering may eventually be possible have recently been heightened by the report of the cloning of a sheep named Dolly. By removing the nucleus from a normal cell of one breed of sheep, and using it to replace the nucleus of an egg obtained from another breed of sheep, a fully functional clone, Dolly, was born following implantation (Wilmut *et al.*, 1997). These same investigators have extended their studies with Dolly and have now produced another sheep, called Polly, that expresses human factor IX in her milk (Schnieke *et al.*, 1997). In both cases, the efficiency of the cloning process was very low but the ability to clone a multicellular individual is itself a dramatic advance and raises the possibility of cloning humans.

Dolly's creation at the hands of scientists has sparked a ferocious debate and even presidential edicts banning research on the cloning of humans in the USA. There is a very real need to be aware of the power of the technology used on a daily basis in the laboratory. In the absence of an ability to ban lethal weapons on a worldwide basis, it seems completely unlikely that there will ever be a consensus to control this type of research. Therefore, the genie is now undoubtedly out of the bag and the uses and abuses of cloning technology depend upon an appreciation of the multicomponent arguments relating to it. Hence, even when even the simplest, most uncontroversial piece of DNA is cloned in the laboratory, the implications of the potential power at work should be clear to each and every one of us.

Conclusion

The remarkable developments in molecular biology in the past few decades are now clearly being translated into clinical medicine. Gene cloning, in particular, is an extremely powerful technique that has become fundamental to many areas of science and clinical medicine. Despite the arguments against the use of gene cloning, it is hoped that this technology will continue to allow the development of new therapies that are superior to currently available treatments.

References

Bagshawe K, Sharma S, Springer C, Antoniw P (1995) Antibody directed prodrug therapy: pilot scale clinical trial. *Tumour Targeting* 1: 1–13.

Boon T, De Plaen E, Lurquin C, *et al.* (1992) Identification of tumour rejection antigens recognised by T lymphocytes. *Cancer Surv* 13: 23–37.

Brady H J M, Miles C G, Pennington D J, Dzierzak E A (1994) Specific ablation of human immunodeficiency virus Tat-expressing cells by conditionally toxic retroviruses. *Proc Natl Acad Sci USA* 91: 365–369.

Brady J, Johnson D, Rubenstein D (1995) *Molecular Medicine*. Oxford: Blackwell Science.

Chester K, Hawkins R (1995) Clinical issues in antibody design. *Trends Biotechnol* 13: 294–300.

Chester K, Hawkins R (1996) Opportunities with phage technology and antibody engineering of fusion proteins. *Advanced Drug Delivery Rev* 22: 303–313.

Deshane J, Loechel F, Conry R, *et al.* (1994) Intracellular single-chain antibody directed against erbB2 and exhibits a selective anti-proliferative effect in erbB2 overexpressing cancer cell lines. *Gene Therapy* 1: 332–337.

Kriegler M (1990) *Gene Transfer and Expression: a Laboratory Manual.* New York, Stockton Press.

McCafferty J, Griffiths A, Winter G, Chiswell D (1990) Phage antibodies: filamentous phage displaying antibody variable domains. *Nature* 348: 552–554.

Maniatis T, Fritsch E F, Sambrook J (1982) *Molecular Cloning: A Laboratory Manual.* Cold Spring Harbor, NY: Cold Spring Harbor Laboratory Press.

Press O, Eary J, Applebaum F, *et al.* (1993) Radiolabelled-antibody therapy of B-cell lymphoma with autologous bone marrow support. *N Engl J Med* 329: 1219–1224.

Robinson H, Torres C (1997) DNA vaccines. *Semin Immunol* 9: 271–283.

Schnieke A E, Kind A J, Ritchie W A, *et al.* (1997) Human factor IX transgenic sheep produced by transfer of nuclei from transfected fetal fibroblasts. *Science* 278: 2130–2133.

Uckun F, Evans W, Forsyth C, *et al.* (1995) Biotherapy of B-cell precursor leukaemia by targeting genistein to CD19-associated tyrosine kinases. *Science* 267: 886–891.

Watt P, Sawaki M, Passaro E (1992) A review of gene transfer techniques. *Am J Surg* 165: 350–355.

Wilmut I, Schnieke A E, McWhir J, *et al.* (1997) Viable offspring derived from fetal and adult mammalian cells. *Nature* 385: 810–813.

4

DNA fingerprinting

Colin D Bingle

One of the most significant advances that underlies the revolution in medical genetics is the ability to visualise directly differences in the sequence of DNA. Such variations in sequence are known as polymorphisms, and they have played major roles in both gene mapping and diagnosis of inherited diseases. Polymorphisms can occur in both exonic and intronic DNA. When found in exonic DNA, polymorphisms may lead to alterations in the amino acid sequence of the protein product of the gene, which may compromise its function, or, if they are present in non-coding regions, they may interfere in the regulation of expression of the RNA

The availability of a variety of restriction enzymes that cleave DNA at specific sites has made possible the identification of polymorphic regions in isolated DNA. These regions can be detected by restriction fragment length polymorphism (RFLP) analysis when the polymorphism involves an enzymatic cleavage site. If the site is altered by the DNA polymorphism then the size of the fragments generated by the specific enzyme cleavage will be altered and can be detected by Southern blotting. Every person carries a significant number of DNA polymorphisms, and this means that no two individuals are identical in molecular make-up apart from a pair of identical twins.

Despite the importance of polymorphisms in human molecular genetics, they are generally only of use if the sequence of the DNA is known and the differences can be identified directly. Molecular tools which are of use in determining variations in regions of DNA that are unknown are therefore of great utility. It is these types of tools that form the basis of the techniques of DNA fingerprinting, and in this chapter I will give a brief outline of the history and development of this important technique as well as an overview of a number of areas in which DNA fingerprinting and related profiling techniques have made a significant impact in medicine and health-related areas. It is not the intention of this overview to provide the reader with practical details of the multitude of fingerprinting techniques that have been developed over the past 10 years.

One of the first steps in the development of DNA fingerprinting techniques was made in 1980 when, quite by chance, Wyman and White (1980) discovered a region of DNA present in a library of random human DNA that was shown to be hypervariable and exhibited multi-allelic variation, i.e. it was repeated at random throughout the genome. During the next few years additional hypervariable regions were identified, and it was found that the variable region in each case consisted of tandem repeats of a short sequence (so-called 'minisatellites'). Allelic differences in the number of such repeats generated polymorphisms that could be detected using restriction enzymes which cut outside of the repeat region and gave rise to alterations in restriction fragment length that could be detected by Southern blotting. The significant breakthrough that gave rise to the techniques of DNA fingerprinting stemmed from the work of Alec Jeffreys and co-workers at the University of Leicester. In studying the human myoglobin gene they identified a minisatellite (Weller *et al.*, 1984) that consisted of four tandem repeats of a 33-base pair (bp) sequence that was related to other characterised human minisatellites (Jeffreys *et al.*, 1985a). When this minisatellite was labelled and used as a probe on Southern blots of human genomic DNA that had been digested with restriction enzymes that cut at sites commonly found in the genome (for example *Hinf* I), multiple bands of hybridising DNA were detected. These bands were of significantly greater size than would be expected from the mean fragment size expected when genomic DNA is cut with these enzymes (0.2–0.4 kb). It was concluded that the larger bands arose from a variable number of repeats in each minisatellite. Using the same probe to screen a human genomic library allowed the identification of a number of related minisatellites containing 3–29 tandem copies of repetitive sequences ranging from 16 to 64 bp in length. Sequence analysis of these repeats identified a consensus sequence that aligned with the original myoglobin gene repeat over a 10- to 15-bp core region. Using a probe to one of these minisatellites (33.15) that comprised 29 almost identical repeats of a 16-bp core, the first so-called 'DNA fingerprints' were produced. In their seminal paper, the authors showed how such probes could be used for paternity analysis and suggested that the technique would find widespread use in segregation analysis, maternity testing and forensic applications. Very rapidly after the original paper was published additional papers showing the use of the technique in these areas were published (Gill *et al.*,1985; Jeffreys *et al.*, 1985b,c, 1986).

Following the identification of these initial minisatellites, it became apparent that some of these regions were exceptionally hypervariable and these could also be used as informative probes on Southern blots (Wong *et al.*, 1987). Because these probes recognise a single locus in genomic DNA, they are known as single-locus probes, in contrast to the original probes, which are known as multiple-locus probes. The fingerprint generated by a single-locus probe provides two bands for analysis on a Southern blot, each band arising from each of the two chromosomal copies in that genomic region (Wong *et al.*, 1987). The very high level of variability found in these regions means that the copy number of repeats that is inherited is often different from the number found in the parents. These single-locus probes are extensively used in forensic applications and generate what is known as a 'DNA profile', a term that is preferable to 'DNA fingerprinting' so as to avoid possible confusion with true fingerprints.

One of the most significant facts with regard to the use of minisatellite probes in DNA fingerprinting and profiling applications (whether they be single- or multiple-locus probes) is that they are simply a representation of an individual's DNA. As they do not normally occur in functional regions of the genome they are not thought to involve regions of DNA that influence a specific phenotype. DNA fingerprinting has now become such a valuable tool in the identification of individuals that a significant number of commercial organisations will provide such services, as a simple search of the Internet will confirm.

Basic techniques of DNA fingerprinting

DNA fingerprinting is based on the detection of regions of digested genomic DNA by Southern blotting. DNA samples are isolated and subjected to digestion by restriction enzymes whose recognition sites appear frequently in the genome. Such enzymes have short recognition sites (typically 4 bp) which are represented in the genome with a greater frequency than those whose recognition sites are greater in length. The digested genomic DNA fragments are resolved by electrophoresis, and the lengths of DNA fragments within the digest that contain the minisatellite regions are increased above the average size for fragments digested with these enzymes and the actual size of the fragments increases as the number of repeats increases. The electrophoresed DNA fragments are then transferred and fixed to a solid membrane support. The membrane is then incubated with a labelled probe to the specific minisatellite region of interest and, where the probe detects an immobilised minisatellite region on the membrane, specific hybridisation occurs. Following washing steps designed to remove any non-specific probe–DNA interactions, the hybridisation pattern can be visualised by the use of either radioactive or non-radioactive detection systems. Such methods give rise to the classic DNA fingerprinting profile that is often likened to the bar code on consumer goods and is thought to be essentially unique to each individual (Jeffreys et al., 1985a). The advent of automated DNA amplification through the process of PCR has also had significant effects on the development and practical uses of DNA fingerprinting/profiling. Many PCR-based DNA profiling techniques have been developed and use, for example, variability in the mitochondrial DNA sequences as well as amplification of minisatellites. Many shorter microsatellites have been identified as well as simple tandem repeats (STRs), regions of multiple repeats of 2–5 bp, which have also been directly used in PCR-based DNA profiling systems (Sutherland and Richards, 1995). PCR-based analysis of such STR regions utilises flanking regions around the repeat regions as the basis of primers for the specific amplification of the inserted region of genomic DNA. Other PCR-based DNA fingerprinting techniques make use of arbitrary sets of oligonucleotide primers in a manner similar to RNA differential display. The advantage of such PCR-based methods is that they are much more amenable to automation and high-throughput screening-based systems. The generation of good-quality DNA fingerprinting relies on the isolation of sufficient quantities of undegraded genomic DNA for the restriction enzyme digestion. For certain applications, for example in forensic science, this may be a problem and, in the case that both quantity and quality of the starting DNA are less than ideal, fingerprinting techniques that rely on the amplification of specific regions may be more informative than those which rely on digestion and Southern blotting of undegraded genomic DNA samples.

Practical applications of DNA fingerprinting

The methods underlying the technique of DNA fingerprinting were originally developed as a tool to investigate hypervariability of DNA within the genome. However, in the original paper describing the technique, Jeffreys et al. (1985a) noted that it could play a major role in a number of areas of genetic medicine and biology. The original report showed that, using a multiple-locus probe on Southern blots, even a single sibship of a first-cousin marriage could be distinguished. One of the significant strengths of DNA fingerprinting is that it allows analysis of individuals without looking at the function and products of specific genes.

Paternity and individual identification by DNA fingerprinting

As already alluded to in the introduction, it is clear that all individuals, with the exception of identical twins, have a unique genetic composition, and it is this uniqueness that makes DNA fingerprinting the best and most conclusive tool for the identification of individuals. Each person inherits half of his or her DNA in equal measure from each biological parent and therefore the DNA fingerprint generated from a child is a composite of the fingerprints generated by the parental DNA. Where samples from both parents are available for analysis, cases of disputed paternity can be resolved beyond statistical doubt. When fingerprinting is performed in all three samples together, all bands found in the child's DNA sample should be found to match bands present in the parental samples. Such clear-cut DNA fingerprinting results were shown in the earliest papers from the Leicester group (Jeffreys *et al.*, 1985a–c).

DNA fingerprinting can also be informative when only one parental sample is available. The earliest example of such a positive identification was made in the case of a Ghanaian boy who attempted to return to the UK with his mother, brother and two sisters after a spell in Ghana. The father's DNA in this case was unavailable and, in any case, the mother was unsure of the paternity of the boy. In this case, using a combination of the DNA fingerprints of the boy, his mother and three siblings (the paternity of whom was not in doubt), it was clearly shown that the boy was a product of the same biological mother and father as the other three siblings (Jeffreys *et al.*, 1985b).

Occasionally due to the hypervariability of some of the regions under study in fingerprinting, new mutations in the hypervariable regions can arise in the child's genomic DNA and are visualised in the DNA fingerprint as a band that is not shared with either parent (Jeffreys *et al.*, 1985b). When such bands are found in the case of disputed paternity (which is very rare) then other parental permutations must be considered. In practice, such a single mutated band identified alongside a large number of bands shared between the parents and the child is normally not considered to be of too great importance.

In addition to its use in simple paternity and immigration cases, DNA fingerprinting has also been used in situations where paternity has been questioned following cases of rape and underaged sex. In these situations it has proved to be possible to use samples from aborted fetuses for the DNA isolation and analysis.

DNA fingerprinting has also crossed into the veterinary world and has been used to confirm the identity and pedigree of a number of species (Buitkamp *et al.*, 1991), including birds and dogs, and has even been used in cases of disputed paternity in the latter (Morton *et al.*, 1987). Additional uses of DNA fingerprinting in the veterinary field include species conservation: in the study of small populations of endangered species the technique can be used to select breeding partners for captive breeding programmes in an effort to maximise genetic diversity in the offspring. Examples include studies performed on wild and captive populations of the Siberian crane (Tokorskaya *et al.*, 1995) as well as captive herds of Speke's gazelle (Butler *et al.*, 1994). DNA fingerprinting has also proved to be an invaluable tool in the tracking of birds and animals stolen from protected sites (Wolfes *et al.*, 1991).

Forensic applications of DNA fingerprinting

Probably the major practical application to which the technique of DNA fingerprinting is applied is in the area of forensic identification. As is the case in the use of fingerprinting for paternity cases, it is the high degree of individuality between profiles that is of such great utility in forensic applications. Forensic samples may be blood spots, hair or other tissues recovered from the scene of a crime or may be blood or tissue samples collected from a range of individual suspects implicated in a particular crime or from a population of potential suspects sampled to exclude particular individuals from an investigation.

The source of the samples provided for forensic DNA fingerprinting studies often dictates the exact methods to be used in the analysis. Tissue samples and blood stains removed from the scene of the crime or from a crime victim may often be suboptimal for the isolation of large quantities of undegraded DNA. Gill *et al.*'s (1985) original application of DNA fingerprinting to forensic applications showed the utility of DNA fingerprinting from blood, semen, hair and vaginal swab samples of different ages. Aged blood and semen stains were found to produce DNA that was somewhat degraded and when these samples were used for classical fingerprinting applications they were shown to generate bands that were less than entirely clear. This finding is important because if the number of bands in a DNA fingerprint is reduced as a result of partial degradation of the initial DNA sample, then the statistical confidence in the result will be reduced.

Thus, in forensic cases, single-locus probes are often used in preference to the classical DNA fingerprinting probes because of the concern that quality of the input DNA sample may be suboptimal. Indeed, the first application of DNA fingerprinting in a British murder case involved the use of single-locus probes (Wong *et al.*, 1987). This case resulted in the release of the original suspect and the capture and conviction of the true murderer. The increased sensitivity of single-locus probes in forensic applications of DNA fingerprinting arises from the fact that, as they detect two bands on the Southern blot, rather than the multiple number found in the classical DNA fingerprint, it is more likely that the probe will detect non-degraded bands in partially degraded genomic DNA isolated from forensic samples.

PCR-based DNA fingerprinting techniques based on analysis of shorter microsatellites and STRs have also been shown to be important tools in forensic applications. Again, the fact that in these situations the DNA may be suboptimal and partially degraded is of less importance than in classical fingerprinting. Furthermore, the power of amplification via PCR makes these techniques rapid to perform and more suited to automation. Such techniques were used recently for the identification of the family of Tsar Nicholas by analysis of DNA extracted from bones from the grave site combined with mitochondrial DNA analysis of samples taken from living relatives, including Prince Philip (Gill *et al.*, 1994).

One area of DNA fingerprinting that has assumed significant importance, particularly with regard to forensic applications, is the absolute confidence with which one can say that a particular fingerprint is unique. This question was the centre of a considerable debate in the late 1980s and early 1990s, when it was shown that DNA fingerprinting patterns were not absolutely independent across loci (Risch and Devlin, 1992), i.e. certain patterns occurred with greater than the statistically predicted frequency in particular ethnic groups, for example differences were found between Hispanics and Caucasians. This observation is particularly important if the probe used for an analysis is found to give different patterns in different ethnic groups. A further concern with regard to the likelihood of a particular DNA fingerprint being shared by two or more individuals is the level of inbreeding within a particular population. Studies have shown that individuals from moderately inbred populations share an increased number of bands in a DNA fingerprint compared to individuals from an outbred population (Bellamy *et al.*, 1991). In this study, the authors suggested that it is therefore important to consider this in forensic cases involving members of an inbred community.

Even allowing for these concerns, it is now widely believed that, if sufficient probes are used, including a combination of both single-locus and multiple-locus probes, and as more information about the distribution of a particular minisatellite within a population is uncovered, the chances of misidentifying a particular individual are statistically remote.

Despite the widespread belief that the evidence generated by DNA fingerprinting in forensic cases can conclusively prove the guilt or innocence of a particular defendant, in some high-profile cases the defendant has been cleared by the jury in the face of apparently overwhelming DNA fingerprinting evidence of guilt. During the recent double murder trial involving the former American football player O J Simpson, large volumes of DNA fingerprinting evidence using multiple loci as probes and DNA samples isolated from blood stains conclusively linked the defendant to the victims. However, the defendant was acquitted owing to doubts concerning the collection of the evidence (Weir, 1995). This case, and others, serves to highlight a fundamental problem in DNA fingerprinting for forensic applications, i.e. the integrity of the evidence must be beyond doubt.

Diagnostic applications of DNA fingerprinting

One area in which DNA fingerprinting has made a significant impact in regard to human health is in diagnosis and epidemiology of micro-biological and viral disease. Just as mammals have hypervariable and minisatellite DNA regions, so do micro-organisms. Analysis of micro-organism hypervariable DNA can detect differences among even closely related strains and is a valuable tool for the medical microbiologist, epidemiologist and virologist (van Belkum, 1994). One of the most extensively studied organisms is *Mycobacterium tuberculosis* (van Soolingen and Hermans, 1995). DNA fingerprinting of *M. tuberculosis* strains is fast replacing the traditional phage-typing methods to distinguish differences in strains.

The initial repetitive element probe used in *M. tuberculosis* DNA fingerprinting, IS6110, was isolated from *M. tuberculosis* (Thierry *et al.*, 1990) and shown to appear in variable copy numbers and in different locations in the chromosome in different clinical isolates (van Soolingen *et al.*, 1991). Additional insertion elements have been isolated from other mycobacteria and have been used as specific diagnostic tools. DNA amplification techniques have also been developed and have been shown to be highly informative and require less input material, thereby reducing the effort and time required for the culture of bacteria from clinical isolates. The availability of such probes has allowed the use of DNA fingerprinting of *M. tuberculosis* strains in a wide variety of epidemiological areas, to study transmission among neighbours, in hospitals and in prisons (van Soolingen and Hermans, 1995) as well as in the investigation of the relative contribution of newly acquired versus reactivated infections in different populations. Large numbers of minisatellite and STR loci have been isolated from a wide range of micro-organisms, viruses and parasites, and these have found uses in the diagnosis and epidemiology of a number of acquired disorders.

Although DNA fingerprinting techniques have become widely used for diagnostic applications, it is still important to accept that there are limitations as to the absolute power of the technique to distinguish between strains (Vaneechoutte and Van Eldere, 1997). In addition, it is also important to recognise the opportunity for the introduction of contamination in laboratories where DNA from specific strains can easily contaminate equipment and reagents. Such problems have been identified where test strains were distributed to a number of laboratories which subsequently mis-identified the samples due to contamination (Vaneechoutte and Van Eldere, 1997).

Confirmation and evaluation of cell sources by DNA fingerprinting

Within both academic and biotechnology laboratories, it is important to be able to monitor and authenticate tissue culture cell lines for use in further experimental procedures. DNA fingerprinting has been used both to show the clonality of such lines and to confirm the cross-contamination of other lines (Thacker *et al.*, 1988; Gilbert *et al.*, 1990; Hay, 1992). Genetic heterogeneity of cell lines derived from different regions of a single tumour has also been studied by DNA fingerprinting (Bettink *et al.*, 1992). In this study, it was shown that genetic differences between individual cell lines derived from a single tumour were similar to differences in the DNA isolated from the region of the tumour mass at the onset of cell line establishment. Similar studies performed on DNA extracted from multiple cell samples at different stages during cell line establishment have shown that somatic mutations occur during the process and, furthermore, these techniques can show that the process of clonal selection occurs during establishment of cell lines (van Helden *et*

al., 1994). DNA fingerprinting has also been used to confirm that differences in cell line responsiveness to anti-tumour drugs over time was not
directly related to significant mutations in the DNA (Ohnishi *et al.*,
1997).

DNA fingerprinting in transplantation biology

The techniques of DNA fingerprinting have been used in a number of
distinct areas related to transplantation biology.

The selection of unrelated donors for bone marrow transplantation
is traditionally performed by the use of serological HLA class typing.
PCR-based fingerprinting has recently been used to improve the selection of donors for such procedures (Martinelli *et al.*, 1996).

The high level of variability seen in fingerprinting has also been har-
nessed to study the success of transplantation; the first report in this area
concerned a patient with a bone marrow transplant (Thein *et al.*, 1986).
Cells and tissues transplanted into an individual will display a unique
DNA profile, and therefore the re-emergence of the recipient's DNA
profile in the blood following transplantation suggests that some of the
recipient's malignant cells survive. This enables early steps to be taken
to review therapy (Weitzel *et al.*, 1988; Dreyfus *et al.*, 1995; Okamoto
et al., 1995).

Fingerprinting techniques have also been applied in solid tissue
transplantations. For example, in some patients receiving donor organs
subsequent lymphoproliferative disease has been shown to be of donor
origin (Armes *et al.*, 1994). There have also been isolated cases in which
DNA fingerprinting has been used to confirm that tumours arising in
organ transplant recipients were the result of transplantation of malignant cells at the time of transplantation.

Conclusion

In this chapter I have attempted to outline the basic principles and some
of the applications of DNA fingerprinting/profiling. It is clear that since
the initial observations of Jeffreys *et al.* in the early 1980s, such techniques have rapidly found uses in many areas of basic science and healthcare. Further advances both in technology and in the understanding of
the role of hypervariable regions of DNA within the genome are likely
to lead to additional applications for DNA profiling in the future.

References

Armes J E, Angus P, Southey M C, *et al.* (1994) Lympoproliferative disease of donor origin arising in patients after orthotopic liver transplantation. *Cancer* 74: 2436–2441.

van Belkum A (1994) DNA fingerprinting of medically important microorganisms by the use of PCR. *Clin Microbiol Rev* 7: 174–184.

Bellamy R J, Inglehearn C F, Jalili I K, *et al.* (1991) Increased band sharing in DNA fingerprints of an inbred human population. *Hum Genet* 87: 341–347.

Bettink S, Wullich B, Christmann A, *et al.* (1992) Genetic heterogeneity of prostatic carcinoma-derived cell lines as emphasized by DNA fingerprinting. *Electrophoresis* 13: 644–646.

Buitkamp J, Ammer H, Geldermann H (1991) DNA fingerprinting in domestic animals. *Electrophoresis* 12: 169–174.

Butler M A, Templeton A R, Read B (1994) DNA fingerprinting in Speke's gazelle: a test for genetic distinctness, and the correlation between relatedness and similarity. *Mol Ecol* 3: 355–361.

Dreyfus F, Ribrag V, Leblond V, *et al.* (1995) Detection of malignant B cells in peripheral blood stem cell collections after chemotherapy in patients with multiple myeloma. *Bone Marrow Transplant* 15: 707–711.

Gilbert D A, Reid Y A, Gail M H, *et al.* (1990) Application of DNA fingerprints for cell-line individualization. *Am J Hum Genet* 47: 499–514.

Gill P, Jeffreys A J, Werrett D J (1985) Forensic application of DNA fingerprints. *Nature* 318: 577–579.

Gill P, Ivanov P L, Kimpton C, *et al.* (1994) Identification of the remains of the Romanov family by DNA analysis. *Nature Genet* 6: 130–135.

Hay R J (1992) Methods for authenticating cell lines. *Dev Biol Stand* 76: 25–37.

van Helden P D, Wiid I J, Hoal-van E G, *et al.* (1994) Detection by DNA fingerprinting of somatic changes during the establishment of a new prostate cell line. *Br J Cancer* 70: 195–198.

Jeffreys A J, Wilson V, Thein S L (1985a) Hypervariable 'minisatellite' regions in human DNA. *Nature* 314: 67–73.

Jeffreys A J, Brookfield J F Y, Semeonoff R (1985b) Positive identification of an immigration test-case using human DNA fingerprints. *Nature* 317: 818–819.

Jeffreys A J, Wilson V, Thein S L (1985c) Individual specific 'fingerprints' of human DNA. *Nature* 316: 76–79.

Jeffreys A J, Wilson V, Thein S L, *et al.* (1986) DNA fingerprints and segregation analysis of multiple markers in human pedigrees. *Am J Hum Genet* 39: 11–24.

Martinelli G, Farabegoli P, Buzzi M, *et al.* (1996) Fingerprinting of HLA class I genes for improved selection of unrelated bone marrow donors. *Eur J Immunogenet* 23: 55–65.

Morton D B, Yaxley R E, Patel I, *et al.* (1987) The use of DNA fingerprinting analysis in identification of the sire. *Vet Rec* 121: 592–593.

Ohnishi Y, Yamamoto N, Ebukuro M, *et al.* (1997) Practical role of genetic profiling and preservation of stock human tumour xenograft lines as a tool in animal experiments for antitumour drug evaluation. *Lab Animal* 31: 169–176.

Okamoto R, Harano H, Matsuzaki M *et al.* (1995) Predicting relapse of chronic myelogenous leukemia after allogenic bone marrow transplantation by bcr-abl mRNA and DNA fingerprinting. *Am J Clin Pathol* 104: 510–516.

Risch N J, Devlin B (1992) On the probability of matching DNA fingerprints. *Science* 255: 717–720.

van Soolingen D, Hermans P M W (1995) Epidemiology of tuberculosis by DNA fingerprinting. *Eur Respir J* 8 (Suppl. 20): 649s–656s.

van Soolingen D, Hermans P M W, de Haas P E W, *et al.* (1991) The occurrence and stability of insertion sequences in *Mycobacterium tuberculosis* complex strains. Evaluation of IS-dependent DNA polymorphisms as a tool in the epidemiology of tuberculosis. *J Clin Microbiol* 29: 2578–2586.

Sutherland G R, Richards R I (1995) Simple tandem repeats and human genetic disease. *Proc Natl Acad Sci USA* 92: 3636–3641.

Thacker J, Webb M B T, Debenham P G (1988) Fingerprinting cell lines: Use of human hypervariable DNA probes to characterize mammalian cell cultures. *Somat Cell Mol Genet* 14: 519–525.

Thein S L, Jeffreys A J, Blacklock H A (1986) Identification of post-transplant cell populations by DNA fingerprint analysis. *Lancet* ii: 37.

Thierry D, Cave M D, Eisenach K D, *et al.* (1990) IS6110, an IS-like element of *M. tuberculosis* complex. *Nucleic Acids Res* 18: 188.

Tokarskaya O N, Petrosyan V G, Kashentseva T, *et al.* (1995) DNA fingerprinting in captive population of the endangered Siberian crane (*Grus leucogeranus*). *Electrophoresis* 16: 1766–1700.

Vaneechoutte M, Van Eldere J (1997) The possibilities and limitations of nucleic acid amplification technology in diagnostic microbiology. *J Med Microbiol* 46: 188–194.

Weir B S (1995) DNA statistics in the Simpson matter. *Nature Genet* 11: 365–368.

Weitzel J N, Horrs J M, Jeffreys A J, *et al.* (1988) Use of a hypervariable minisatellite DNA probe (33.15) for evaluating engraftment two or more years after bone marrow transplantation for aplastic anaemia. *Br J Haematol* 70: 91–97.

Weller P, Jeffreys A J, Wilson V, *et al.* (1984) Organization of the human myoglobin gene. *EMBO J* 3: 439–446.

Wolfes R, Mathe, J, Seitz A (1991) Forensics of birds of prey by DNA fingerprinting with ^{32}P-labelled oligonucleotide probes. *Electrophoresis* 12: 175–180.

Wong Z, Wilson V, Patel I, *et al.* (1987) Characterization of a panel of highly variable minisatellites cloned from human DNA. *Ann Hum Genet* 51: 269–288.

Wyman A, White R (1980) A highly polymorphic locus in human DNA. *Proc Natl Acad Sci USA* 77: 6754–6758.

5

The polymerase chain reaction (PCR): general applications and potential for clinical use

Gavin Brooks

The polymerase chain reaction, or PCR, is one of the most significant and fundamental scientific discoveries of recent times and has proved to be an indispensable analytical tool for any discipline interested in analysing DNA or mutations in DNA. The PCR was first described in the mid-1980s (Saiki *et al.*, 1985), although it was based on a concept first proposed almost 15 years earlier (Kleppe *et al.*, 1971; Panet and Khorana, 1974). After a few refinements (Mullis and Faloona, 1987; Saiki *et al.*, 1988), this technique has revolutionised almost every field of biological and clinical research and has rapidly become established as one of the most widely used molecular biological techniques available because it is a rapid, inexpensive and simple method for the exponential amplification of very small amounts of DNA into much larger amounts. Since its discovery, the PCR has been used in numerous applications, and its global significance was highlighted in 1993 when the original discoverer, Dr Kary B Mullis, was awarded the Nobel Prize for Chemistry in recognition of the extraordinary impact of PCR technology on scientific research generally. In recent years, the potential uses of the PCR have led to the growth of a multimillion pound industry producing products to supply the rapidly expanding market as this now commonplace technique is adapted to solve problems in all fields of science and clinical medicine. In medicine, for example, the PCR has had a major impact on diagnosis and screening of genetic diseases and cancer and has been used for the rapid detection of fastidious or slow-growing micro-organisms and viruses, e.g. mycobacteria and human immunodeficiency virus (HIV).

This chapter will describe the basic principles of the PCR and discuss how it is being used for biomedical research and in routine screening procedures.

Replication of DNA – the molecule of life

Until the advent of the PCR, the manipulation of DNA, and in particular specific genes or sequences, was hindered by the lack of availability of a rapid and simple method of analysis. Thus, until recently, it was not easy to purify a specific sequence of DNA from a large mixture of sequences, even if the location of that sequence in the DNA was known. Furthermore, detection of a given sequence in a sample of DNA was often a problem because most techniques for studying DNA are relatively insensitive, require large amounts of starting material and are time-consuming. The availability of the PCR has solved all of these problems and enables the simple and rapid manipulation of DNA. The original PCR protocol (Saiki *et al.*, 1985) was based on a very simple idea, the mechanics of which had been around for millions of years in the form of normal cell division. Every time a cell divides, it is required to duplicate itself entirely, including its DNA content. By harnessing a modified version of this process *in vitro*, it has become possible to amplify a specific sequence of DNA in large quantities. Although DNA replication in a cell is a very complicated process – with a vast number of proteins interacting together to produce the final duplicated DNA – the essential components are few. These components are the original DNA to be copied; the three enzymes DNA helicase, RNA primase and DNA-dependent DNA polymerase; and the four nucleotide triphosphates (dNTPs), guanosine (G), cytosine (C), adenosine (A) and thymidine (T). In mammals, DNA replication proceeds as follows (Figure 5.1). The enzyme DNA helicase attaches to double-stranded DNA and separates the two strands at fairly random points. RNA primase then attaches to either one of the strands of DNA and produces a short 10-bp strand of RNA complementary to the DNA strand to which it binds. The original strand of DNA is known as the template and the RNA strand is known as the primer since it serves as a starting point for the action of the third enzyme, DNA-dependent DNA polymerase. This enzyme produces an exact complementary copy of the template DNA using the original DNA strand as a template, the short RNA strand as a primer for DNA elongation and the free dNTPs as the building blocks for the new DNA strand. The process of copying the DNA strand continues until the DNA-dependent DNA polymerase enzyme reaches the end of the template strand or until it reaches the beginning of another replication point. This process will occur at many places throughout the genome and on *both* DNA strands. DNA replication will continue until both strands have been replicated completely, thus leaving the cell with two exact

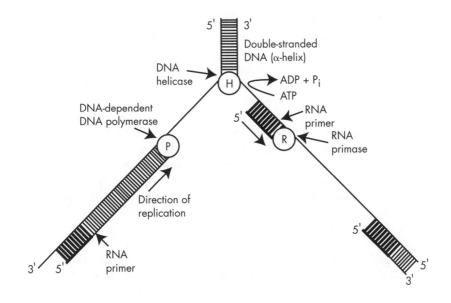

Figure 5.1   Replication of DNA in mammalian cells showing the sites of action of the enzymes DNA helicase, DNA-dependent DNA polymerase and RNA primase.

copies of its original DNA. In reality, this physiological process is far more complicated and is too intricate to use as a standard technique for replicating DNA in the laboratory. Furthermore, if the process was mimicked in a test tube, the amount of DNA produced would be only twice the amount of starting material, which would not produce sufficient material for analysis. Most importantly, this approach would not provide the specificity required – for example to enhance the production of one specific gene. Despite these apparent drawbacks, the process has been used to our advantage by utilising the relatively simple procedure of the PCR.

Principles of PCR technology

It now is possible to mimic cellular DNA replication in a test tube by utilising the following basic concepts:

1   DNA is composed of two long strands of nucleotides which are exact complementary copies of each other (in which G will bind to C and T will bind to

A). These strands are held together by non-covalent hydrogen bonds between the complementary nucleotides in each strand. If the temperature of the DNA is raised to more than 90°C, the hydrogen bonds will break and the two strands will separate (a procedure known as denaturation or melting) in a similar manner to the effects of the DNA helicase enzyme. Thus, heating removes the requirement for this enzyme under laboratory conditions.

2 Just as DNA strands can be separated by increased temperatures, complementary sequences of DNA will join (or anneal) to each other when temperatures fall below a specific level (generally 55–65°C).

3 It now is relatively easy and inexpensive to synthesise short (between 15 and 50 bp), specific lengths of DNA (oligonucleotides) of any specific sequence. These oligonucleotides then can be annealed to the complementary sequence of the target DNA in a test tube, thereby removing the requirement for the enzyme RNA primase. In addition, this results in replication of very specific portions of the sample DNA simply by synthesising the correct oligonucleotide primers to the sequence of interest rather than having a random replication of DNA.

4 DNA-dependent DNA polymerase will replicate DNA strands specifically in a 5′ to 3′ direction (see Figure 5.1) using a short double-stranded sequence as a starting or priming site and single-stranded DNA as a template.

5 The bacterial enzyme *Taq* DNA polymerase (Kaledin *et al*., 1982) has a similar function to normal mammalian DNA polymerases. This enzyme was isolated originally from the bacterium *Thermus aquaticus*, which grows in the hot springs of Yellowstone National Park (Chien *et al*., 1976). Following analysis of this organism, many of the enzymes present in *T. aquaticus* were found to be heat stable. The optimal temperature for activity of purified *Taq* DNA polymerase was found to be 72°C, although it can withstand temperatures as high as 99°C and still retain enzymatic activity. The isolation of this enzyme was one of the major advances which enabled the development of the PCR as a routine technique, since before its discovery only heat-labile enzymes were available, and these were obviously destroyed by the denaturation step of the reaction (i.e. heating to 99°C). A further advantage of using *Taq* DNA polymerase is the much higher optimal temperature of activity of the enzyme. Thus, the temperature of the PCR reaction does not need to fall below the annealing temperature at any stage as *Taq* DNA polymerase requires a much higher temperature for optimal activation than mammalian DNA polymerases, thereby greatly reducing problems with primer mismatch, i.e. the process where two non-complementary DNA sequences anneal to each other leading to an incorrect DNA sequence being produced.

Basic procedure for a successful PCR reaction

The PCR uses the combination of the above five basic principles to replicate and amplify a specific DNA sequence in a PCR reaction such that a single copy of a DNA sequence can be amplified to produce millions of copies within a matter of hours. Essentially, the process has two primary phases:

1   a screening phase that occurs during the first few cycles in which the desired DNA fragment is selected by specific primer binding; and
2   an amplification phase that occurs during subsequent cycles in which the copy number of the desired DNA fragment increases exponentially.

A typical PCR reaction is carried out as shown in Figure 5.2.

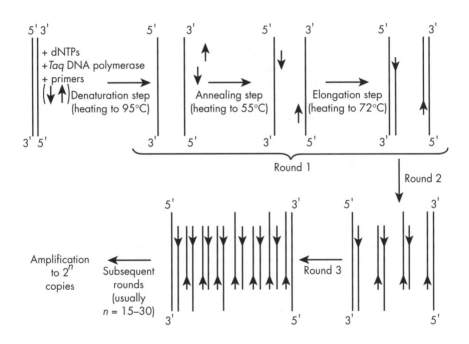

Figure 5.2   The polymerase chain reaction. The process is shown in detail for the first round of amplification. Subsequent rounds have identical steps.

1   The sample DNA (as little as 10 ng of total genomic DNA or 1 pg of plasmid DNA), dNTPs, *Taq* DNA polymerase and primers created to specific sequences at the two ends (but to opposite strands) of the DNA sequence of interest are mixed in a buffered solution (pH 8.4) and heated to 90–95°C in a thermocycler for 1 minute. This leads to denaturation of the double-stranded DNA into two single strands.

2   The temperature then is lowered to approximately 55°C for 1 minute, which enables the primers to anneal specifically to the complementary sequences to which they were constructed without enabling them to anneal to incorrect, non-specific sequences. As shown in Figure 5.2, each of the oligonucleotide primers anneals to a different DNA strand at either end of the sequence of interest. Since, by definition, replication always occurs in the 5′ to 3′ direction on either DNA strand, the area of interest on both template strands is replicated.

3   The temperature then is increased to 72°C for 2 minutes to permit the *Taq* DNA polymerase enzyme to replicate (polymerise) the new strand by extending the primer sequence, using the original DNA strand as a template. This results in one complementary copy of the DNA sequence being produced.

4   Further copies of the sequence are produced by repeating the processes described in steps 1–3 between 15 and 30 times, which results in an exponential increase in the number of copies of DNA produced in the order of $S \times 2^n$, where S is the starting amount of a sample DNA and n is the number of rounds of replication. Thus, even 10 rounds of replication can lead to a 2^{10} or a 1024-fold amplification of the original DNA sample. In general, 25–35 cycles are sufficient to produce 100 ng to 1 μg of a 1-kb single-copy human sequence using 50 ng of starting genomic DNA. In order to maximise the chances of a successful outcome, it is important that the reaction conditions during the first few cycles are designed to minimise the possibility of primers initiating an extension reaction from any part of the template mixture that is not the desired DNA sequence. Similarly, the reaction conditions used after the first few cycles should be those that permit all newly synthesised molecules to be perfectly replicated at high efficiency so they double in number after each cycle.

5   The results of the PCR reaction can be observed in a number of ways depending upon the exact technique being used, but the easiest method is to separate the DNA fragments by electrophoresis in an agarose gel containing the fluorescent dye ethidium bromide (which stains nucleic acids). Stained bands then can be visualised under an ultraviolet light source (Figure 5.3). A preliminary identification of the PCR product can be made by comparison of the size of the PCR product (calculated from size markers run on the same gel; see Figure 5.3) with that predicted from the DNA sequence of interest.

It is important to stress that no one individual protocol will be optimal for all PCR reactions, nor will any single, simple set of variables to be optimised necessarily produce a functionary protocol for a specific case. However, the basic PCR procedure achieves two very useful objectives: firstly, it can increase the amount of sample DNA considerably in a relatively short period of time; and, secondly, and perhaps more importantly, it can be used to isolate a specific region or sequence of DNA from a large amount of surrounding or contaminating DNA. This means, for example, that from a very small tissue sample – perhaps containing only

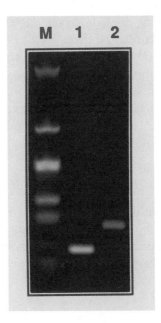

Figure 5.3 Agarose gel electrophoresis showing typical results from a PCR reaction. Lane 1 shows amplification of a 241-bp fragment from a deletion mutant of the glyceraldehyde dehydrogenase (GAPDH) gene, whereas lane 2 shows the normal GAPDH gene as a 396-bp fragment amplified using the same primers as in lane 1. M denotes pGEM size markers.

a few cells or even a single cell – it is theoretically possible to amplify and isolate a specific gene or DNA sequence for analysis.

Advantages and disadvantages of the PCR

In common with most *in vitro* techniques, the PCR produces a number of advantages and disadvantages for the user, as outlined below.

Advantages of the PCR

Specificity

The PCR is highly specific and can identify accurately even a single base pair mutation in a DNA sequence containing thousands of base pairs.

The degree of specificity does, however, depend upon the choice of primers used in the reaction, and these need to be exact or nearly exact matches for the desired DNA sequence to be amplified. Primers should also have virtually no homology to other sequences in the template mixture. In general, primers that are 18 or more nucleotides in length should be unique within a complex eukaryotic genome, whereas primers as short as 10 nucleotides are likely to be unique for any purified cloned DNA fragment.

Rapidity

Results are possible within hours with this method (e.g. a 30-cycle amplification of a 200-bp DNA sequence can be completed within 3 hours), whereas conventional techniques require many days or even weeks. Also, large numbers of samples can be analysed at the same time.

Versatility

The basic technique can be adapted in a number of ways. For example, although the 3′ end of a primer needs to be very specific, there is a certain amount of adaptability in the rest of the primer. Thus, by reducing the reaction stringency, a primer can be used to amplify slightly differing sequences. Also the 5′ end of the primer can actually be totally different from the sample sequence and so it is possible to add on sequences to the ends of a PCR product. This method is used for introducing mutations into genes.

Ease of use

Once the reactants have been added together, all subsequent steps are fully automated. The reaction tube is placed into a thermocycler, which is programmed to complete the required number of cycles. Any individual with laboratory training and who has access to this relatively inexpensive (approximately £3000) piece of equipment can carry out a PCR.

Quantity

It is possible to analyse a large number of samples at one time or to analyse a single sample for the presence of multiple genes or mutations simply by adding multiple primer pairs to the same sample tube. This is obviously dependent upon the DNA products being of sufficiently different sizes to be separated by gel electrophoresis and subsequently detected (Figure 5.3).

Purity of sample

The PCR is tolerant of poor-quality template DNA since partially degraded samples can be used to generate results when other analytical techniques would be useless. The template DNA can originate from a variety of sources, including intact tissue specimens, blood and serum samples, nucleic acids from archival specimens, biopsy specimens embedded in paraffin, cloned DNA fragments or even PCR products themselves.

Disadvantages of the PCR

Identity of the DNA sequence

The DNA sequence of interest must be partly known or at least be relatively well predicted. However, since it generally is possible to predict the sequence of a gene of interest, or at least a part of it, from homologous genes with similar activities, this problem can usually be overcome. From such predictions it is possible to produce 'degenerate primers', which are a mixture of oligonucleotide primers each with one of the possible sequences for that gene and which should be able to amplify the sequence of interest.

Size of sequence

There is a limit to the length of sequence that can be effectively amplified using the PCR. Generally, this is in the region of about 0.1–3 kb, although larger fragments (up to 35 kb) can be obtained under ideal conditions. The problem arises because *Taq* DNA polymerase is not normally required to copy such long lengths of DNA in the bacterial cell and tends to 'fall off' the DNA strand being copied if substrate dNTPs become depleted or if conditions are not ideal. However, as the PCR is generally not used for isolating long stretches of genomic DNA, this usually does not pose a major problem.

Number of cycles

If too many cycles are carried out when analysing very small quantities of DNA, such as from a single cell, the primers and dNTP levels may become limiting or the *Taq* DNA polymerase may lose its activity, resulting in insufficient amplification. To overcome this problem, a small quantity of the first reaction can be used as a template for a second PCR. It is imperative that the reaction is stopped before the major product becomes saturated and can no longer increase exponentially since any contaminating molecules will continue to increase exponentially.

Contaminating DNA

The slightest trace of contamination in any of the solutions or the sample DNA with foreign DNA can lead to false-positive results, and so suitable positive and negative controls should be used and extreme cleanliness must be maintained at all times. Contamination is a serious concern in PCR reactions and must be avoided at all costs. To prevent contamination of samples by previously amplified products, considerable care should be exercised as follows:

1   Micropipettes that are used only for the preparation of PCR reaction mixtures should be employed in addition to the use of a designated PCR workstation that is set apart from the rest of the laboratory.
2   Products obtained from completed amplifications should be handled with a separate set of pipettes located in a different part of the laboratory.
3   The primary concern in any PCR amplification is 'carryover' of amplified target DNA to unamplified reaction mixtures. Thus, suitable negative control reactions (i.e. complete reaction mixtures lacking template DNA) should be included in each experiment as an assay for overt contamination.
4   Internal standards always should be included in each assay to control for the rate of amplification, which can fluctuate from sample to sample depending upon the presence of polymerase inhibitors.

Non-specific amplification

Serious problems can occur when the primers bind to closely related DNA sequences in the sample, leading to the wrong sequence being amplified. Such problems can generally be overcome either by raising the annealing temperature of the target DNA and/or by altering the reaction conditions to increase the stringency. In the worst cases, changing the primer sequences to a more specific area may be required.

Recent refinements to the PCR amplification procedure

A number of improvements have recently been made to the basic PCR reaction that have increased the versatility of the technique such that the dynamic balance is shifted towards the desired DNA product. These are described below.

Hot-start PCR

This involves starting the reaction at a high temperature to avoid problems arising from primers annealing to the wrong sequences, which can occur under the low-stringency conditions that are present during the initial heating up of the reactants from room temperature to the temperature required for the first denaturation step. Thus, problems associated with amplification of false positives will be minimised.

Booster PCR

This approach uses lower primer concentrations during the first few cycles to minimise priming from the wrong direction. This is followed by 'boosting' the primer concentration to promote exponential amplification of the already enriched desired DNA template.

Touchdown PCR

This reaction involves reducing the annealing temperature gradually, especially during the first few cycles, such that the initial priming reactions will occur only on DNA sequences with perfect homology to the primers.

Nested PCR

This approach is used to improve the sensitivity and specificity of both DNA and RNA amplification when dealing with poor-quality or low-copy-number nucleic acid template. Nested PCR is especially useful for analysing archival material from paraffin-embedded tissue, for the detection of very rare sequences and for studying persistent viral infections (Jackson *et al.*, 1991). The nested PCR process uses two consecutive PCR reactions, each usually involving 25 cycles of amplification. The first PCR uses an external pair of primers while the second contains two 'nested' primers that are internal to the first primer pair.

Alternatively, a single nested primer can be used. The largest fragment produced from the first reaction (using the outermost primers) serves as a template for the second PCR (using the nested primers). The result is effectively 50 cycles of amplification of the fragment flanked by the nested primer pair. It has been reported that this approach is up to 1000 times more sensitive than 50 cycles of standard PCR (Jackson *et al.*, 1991).

Uses of the PCR in research and clinical diagnosis

Since its discovery, the potential of the PCR has been realised both in basic research and in clinical medicine, and many applications of the technique have significant commercial potential. Not surprisingly, therefore, the PCR process and polymerase enzymes that drive the reaction are the subjects of various patents, now held by Hoffman-La Roche. Some of the current uses of this revolutionary technique are described below (see also Table 5.1).

Table 5.1   Uses of the polymerase chain reaction

Basic science
Identification of new genes and gene families
Mutagenesis studies
Analysis of mRNA expression
Archaeological investigations
DNA cloning and screening of DNA clones
DNA sequencing
Gene mapping, e.g. the Human Genome Project

Clinical medicine
Infectious disease screening
HIV detection
Prenatal diagnosis
Sex determination
Mutational analysis in inherited disease
Detection of abnormalities in haematological diseases
Detection of oncogenes and tumour-suppressor gene mutations in malignant and premalignant diseases
Forensic pathology
HLA subtyping
Detection of susceptibility to cardiovascular disease

Uses of the PCR in research

Identification of new genes

The PCR has been used efficiently to find rare genes from cDNA libraries (i.e. a collection of all genes in a cell or tissue) and to identify complex related gene families (McPherson *et al.*, 1991; Ross and Chien, 1991).

Mutagenesis of DNA sequences

Alterations in the sequence of DNA, e.g. replacement of one nucleotide with another, can be achieved rapidly by the PCR. Such mutated sequences can be used to determine their effects on, for example, growth of cells or for monitoring the ability of the sequence to induce cancer.

Molecular archaeology

The PCR enables the amplification of DNA from archival material, e.g. from preserved surgical specimens. Such specimens are often of pathological interest, having been obtained from unusual or rare clinical conditions, and it may be of interest to study their nucleic acid composition.

Analysis of messenger RNA (mRNA)

The PCR can be used quantitatively to measure the levels of specific mRNAs in different cell populations or tissues or in the same tissue at different developmental stages by a technique called reverse transcription PCR (RT-PCR). In this reaction, the mRNA is first reverse transcribed into complementary DNA (cDNA), which then is subjected to conventional PCR amplification. The amount of mRNA of interest is compared with the amount of amplified mRNA from a control gene (which produces a different-sized band by electrophoresis) in the same reaction. This method is particularly useful when analysing low-abundance mRNAs or when limited amounts of material are available (McPherson *et al.*, 1991).

Uses of the PCR in clinical medicine

Although originally devised as a technique for laboratory research, the versatility of the PCR has led to its development for use in a wide variety of clinical applications. Such analyses were not possible before the advent of the PCR, required large samples to work with or simply were less efficient than PCR amplification in terms of time and sensitivity. Listed below are a few of the many uses to which the PCR is applied currently in clinical medicine.

Diagnosis of inherited diseases

The PCR has revolutionised human genetics by increasing the speed and sensitivity of analysis. In many inherited diseases it is necessary to detect a single base pair difference between the normal and mutated gene, and a number of procedures based on the PCR are now available for the routine detection of known mutations. For example, assays based on this technique now permit presymptomatic or antenatal diagnosis of inherited diseases such as Duchenne muscular dystrophy, fragile X syndrome, Lesch–Nyhan syndrome, Tay–Sachs disease and Kennedy disease (McPherson et al., 1991; Harper, 1996). The approach is also used clinically to detect all of the four common mutations which cause cystic fibrosis (Markham, 1993). Direct diagnosis by the PCR is used to screen essential regions of the factor IX gene for mutations which lead to haemophilia B, and DNA from relatives has been analysed to detect possible carriers of this inherited disease (McPherson et al., 1991).

Infectious disease screening

It is often important clinically to be able to detect incredibly low levels of a particular sequence of DNA in patient samples. An example of this is the detection of HIV, a virus that is not detectable by conventional methods in the circulation but which is detectable by the PCR using specific oligonucleotide primers to the viral DNA. This is now used on a regular basis as a rapid and sensitive method for HIV screening in genitourinary clinics and provides results more rapidly than the conventional method of immunological screening (Markham, 1993). The PCR also has been used to detect the measles virus RNA in brain biopsy specimens from patients with subacute sclerosing panencephalitis (Markham, 1993) and for the detection of herpesvirus DNA in the aqueous humour of uveitis patients, in whom it has been used for confirmation of the clinical diagnosis of viral uveitis (Yamamoto et al., 1996). The PCR has also been employed in the diagnosis of upper respiratory tract infections caused by certain adenoviruses, e.g. pharyngoconjunctival fever and pneumonia (throat swabs are taken and primers derived from the hexon region DNA sequences of endemic adenovirus serotypes 2 and 5 are used to amplify diagnostic sequences) (Morris et al., 1996), and sexually transmitted diseases (urine specimens can be screened for the presence of *Chlamydia trachomatis* infection using a commercial PCR assay – Amplicor *C. trachomatis* test, Roche Diagnostic Systems Inc., Branchburg, NJ, USA) (Quinn *et al.*, 1996). In these cases, the PCR serves as a sensitive and specific non-invasive diagnostic assay, although currently it is relatively expensive since each specimen costs more than US$100 to process and test results take 3–4 days as nucleic acids have to be extracted from the specimen prior to PCR amplification (Stapleton, 1996). Recently, it has been suggested that the PCR could be used to detect sexually transmitted diseases in vaginal washes obtained from prepubertal girls for the purpose of providing evidence for sexual abuse in children (Embree *et al.*, 1996) and to diagnose Lyme disease, for which a simple, nested PCR assay has been developed based on the amplification of the outer surface protein A (OspA) gene fragment of *Borrelia burgdorferi*. This sensitive assay enables the detection of as few as five spirochaetes per millilitre of vehicle and is particularly useful because in Lyme disease there is no serological response in early, partially treated and/or seronegative chronic disease (Mouritsen *et al.*, 1996).

Forensic examination

The PCR technique is used regularly by forensic laboratories to detect and identify blood, tissue and hair samples, semen stains and even cigarette butts from crime scenes where only minuscule amounts of sample are available. It has been estimated that only 30 μl of semen (5–10 μg of DNA) or a 2.5-mm^2 spot of blood (0.5–1 μg of DNA) is required for an accurate PCR analysis for identification purposes (McPherson *et al.*, 1991). More recently, it has been reported that the PCR can be used to identify criminals from DNA in fingerprints left on objects even after the prints have been wiped off and also from DNA deposited inside gloves worn by criminals (Anderson, 1997). Indeed, researchers at the Victoria Forensic Science Centre in Melbourne, Australia, have identified individuals from the tiny quantities of DNA in their fingerprints such that a successful identification could be made from as little as 0.5 ng of material.

Sex determination and prenatal screening

Prenatal sex determination is often required in families with a history of inherited sex-linked diseases, e.g. haemophilia. In such cases, chorionic villus samples are ideal for fetal sexing in the first trimester of pregnancy, and 5 mg of tissue (1–3 μg of DNA) is all that is required. Fetal sexing and fetal diagnostic testing can be carried out using amniotic fluid samples since the sensitivity of the PCR makes it possible to amplify sequences from fetal cells found in amniotic fluid. Prenatal screening is currently used to check for the presence of sickle cell anaemia, thalassaemia and Duchenne muscular dystrophy (Ross and Chien, 1991). The ability to detect negligible amounts (a few molecules) of DNA is also essential for preimplantation diagnosis in *in vitro* fertilisation clinics, and a method utilising PCR technology is currently in use (Markham, 1993). Furthermore, the method can be used to determine quickly, from a variety of tissue samples, whether a fetus is male (McPherson *et al.*, 1991). In this approach, primers which flank part of the Y chromosome are used in a standard PCR amplification procedure. The testing of a female sample will obviously produce negative results, and so it is imperative that suitable controls are run to ascertain the accuracy of the technique. Although this method is relatively straightforward, the greater sensitivity afforded by PCR can cause problems as a result of possible contamination from maternal cells in the fluid, which could result in a misdiagnosis. The PCR also has been used to detect Batten's disease in the fetus (Munroe *et al.*, 1996). This is the most common progressive encephalopathy of childhood in Western countries and is due, in more than 80% of cases, to a major 1-kb deletion in the genome. Termination of pregnancy followed the positive diagnosis of Batten's disease by PCR in a fetus in Finland recently (Munroe *et al.*, 1996).

HLA subtyping

Hospital haematology units are now using PCR analysis routinely to screen patients for their HLA molecular subtype. Clinicians are now attempting to develop tests using this subtyping procedure to predict patients at risk of developing insulin-dependent diabetes mellitus (Markham, 1993).

Susceptibility to cardiovascular disease

Genetic mutations that predispose individuals to myocardial infarction [a mutation in the angiotensin-converting enzyme (ACE) gene] or hypertension (a mutation in the angiotensinogen gene) have recently been identified. Clinicians now are pushing for large population screening programmes to detect these mutations so that affected individuals can be counselled and advised to change their lifestyles or eating habits accordingly.

In another procedure, genomic DNA obtained from patients' white blood cells has been tested by the PCR for the presence of point mutations in the apolipoprotein CII gene and the low-density lipoprotein (LDL) receptor (Ross and Chien, 1991), both of which are indicators of atherosclerosis.

Susceptibility to cancer

Exfoliative cytology specimens can be collected by washing, scraping or aspiration techniques. These specimens could include cells found in urine, sputum, pleural effusions or from uterine cervix. The analysis of such specimens by the PCR is being used clinically to obtain a rapid indication of the presence of neoplastic disease, e.g. following cervical smear testing (McPherson et al., 1991). In other instances, the PCR has been used in the identification of presurgical lymph node metastases in melanoma patients (Schwurzer-Voit et al., 1996) and to confirm diagnosis of acute promyelocytic leukaemia and chronic myelogenous leukaemia by detecting specific chromosomal translocations (Drexler et al., 1995; Wujcik, 1996). The technique has also been used to monitor response of these diseases to chemotherapeutic agents and to predict disease progression. Recently, researchers at the Columbia Presbyterian Medical Center in New York City have patented a new test for thyroid cancer (Lewis, 1997). This form of cancer is frequently asymptomatic, and follow-up assessment of residual disease can be very uncomfortable because patients are required to stop taking thyroid hormone supplements temporarily, which leads to a distressing hypothyroid state. The newly developed test uses RT-PCR to detect thyroglobulin mRNA in patients' blood (Lewis, 1997). Since thyroglobulin is thyroid cell specific, any mRNA detected in blood is indicative of metastatic disease. Although this test is not quantitative and requires refinement, it does serve as a valuable adjunct to more conventional means of diagnosis. Other uses of the PCR in detecting cancers include the detection of T-cell receptor delta gene rearrangements as a measure of minimal residual disease in acute lymphoblastic leukaemia and non-Hodgkin's lymphoma (Chan et al., 1996) and for monitoring secondary alveolar rhabdomyosarcomas that have disseminated to the bone marrow or peripheral blood (Kelly et al., 1996).

Despite the potential importance of the PCR as a rapid detection method for cancers, the technique essentially remains in its experimental stages for the detection of covert disease. Clinicians still have to rely on less sensitive but currently more acceptable forms of diagnosis, e.g. morphology, immunophenotyping and cytogenetics. However, the PCR is useful as an additional diagnostic tool and is likely to become invaluable in the future for staging tumours, monitoring the effects of therapy on the progression of the disease and for post-therapy follow-up.

Future potential

As detailed above, there already are many applications in which the PCR is being used both in research and in the clinic. However, it is without doubt that more specific uses for this versatile technique will arise. Three areas in which PCR probably will be utilised routinely in the near future are non-invasive fetal diagnosis, early detection of cancer and cardio-vascular medicine.

Non-invasive fetal diagnosis

There has been a great deal of concern among clinicians and expectant mothers alike that invasive techniques for fetal diagnosis, e.g. amnio-centesis and chorionic villus sampling, can cause harm to the unborn fetus, e.g. by increasing the risk of miscarriage. However, in 1989 it was shown that it was possible to detect a Y chromosome-specific product from an enriched fetal cell preparation obtained from the peripheral blood of pregnant women carrying a male fetus (Lo *et al.*, 1989). It has been estimated that there are fewer than 10 000 fetal nucleated erythro-cytes present in 20 ml of maternal blood, thus making analysis difficult owing to maternal cell contamination. However, attempts are being made to enrich for fetal cells (using specific antibodies), which would reduce the problems of maternal DNA contamination. If this technique can be optimised in the future, it could easily be used to apply the full range of diagnoses for chromosomal abnormalities associated with birth defects, e.g. trisomy of chromosome 21 (Down's syndrome). This would possibly avoid the need for invasive techniques entirely or at least limit them to those cases requiring an additional confirmatory diagnosis.

Early detection of cancer

The early detection of cancer is important clinically for a good prognosis in virtually all types of cancers, and curative surgery is also likely to be more successful, e.g. in colon cancer. Unfortunately, it is often difficult to obtain samples in a form that can be used in a screening programme even though a number of gene mutations have now been identified as being linked to precancerous cells. However, using the PCR, it may be possible to detect changes in cellular DNA from a very small number of cells. For example, mutations in the p53 gene have been shown to be indicative of developing bladder cancer. Such cancerous cells can be detected by analysis of shed cells present in patients' urine samples (Sidransky *et al.*, 1991). Likewise, it is possible by the PCR to detect premalignant changes in the gastrointestinal tract, by testing DNA from faecal samples for shed intestinal cells containing so-called tumour-suppressor gene mutations (Sidransky *et al.*, 1992). Patients at high risk of disease then could be selected for colonoscopy and any further treatment. It remains to be shown in this instance, however, whether the PCR approach would be more advantageous than the current practise of faecal occult testing. In addition, the PCR could be used for detecting the presence of gastric *Helicobacter pylori* infection (an indicator of gastric malignancy) by assessing stool samples, thereby avoiding the need for invasive endoscopic examination of the patient. Finally, the identification of genes that are associated with tumour spread or metastases, e.g. *nm23* in melanoma, may make it possible to screen patients who have been newly diagnosed with primary melanoma for potentially metastatic cells in the circulation (Pittman *et al.*, 1991).

Cardiovascular medicine

Molecular studies of genetic/acquired cardiac diseases have been hampered by the inability to clone and characterise the genes that are aberrantly expressed in the myocardium in a range of pathological states, e.g. familial cardiomyopathy. However, the ability to amplify genetic material in small numbers of myocardial cells may lead to new horizons in clinical cardiovascular medicine. The PCR should enable construction of cDNA libraries from cardiac biopsy specimens and lead to the subsequent molecular characterisation of human cardiac disorders (Ross and Chien, 1991).

Conclusions and summary

The PCR is unique as new techniques go in terms of the speed with which it has been embraced by non-experts in most areas of the biological sciences, including medicine, and during the past 5 years it has become probably the most widely used single technique. The reasons for this are the rapidity, sensitivity and specificity of the method coupled with the fact that the equipment is inexpensive and running costs are low. It is clear that the PCR is of immense use to both research and clinical workers in all fields and already is used for the routine identification of new genes and mutations in many cell types as well as in the diagnosis of both genetic and infectious diseases within many hospital departments. The simplicity and ease of use of the technique enables investigations or diagnoses on a large scale with many more samples than it would normally be possible to screen by conventional methods. It is feasible that the sequencing of the entire human genome could be achieved by the end of the decade using PCR technology. The achievement of this long-term goal should enable the causes of many more genetic diseases to be identified.

References

Anderson I (1997) The dabs that won't wipe clean. *New Scientist* 11, 21 June.

Chan D W, Liang R, Kwong Y L, Chan V (1996) Detection of T-cell delta gene rearrangement in T-cell malignancies by clonal specific polymerase chain reaction and its application to detect minimal residual disease. *Am J Hematol* 52: 171–177.

Chien A, Edgar D B, Trela J M (1976) Deoxyribonucleic acid polymerase from the extreme thermophile *Thermus aquaticus*. *J Bacteriol* 127: 1550–1557.

Drexler H G, Borkhardt A, Janssen J W (1995) Detection of chromosomal translocations in leukemia–lymphoma cells by polymerase chain reaction. *Leukemia Lymphoma* 19: 359–380.

Embree J E, Lindsay D, Williams T, *et al.* (1996) Acceptability and usefulness of vaginal washes in premenarcheal girls as a diagnostic procedure for sexually transmitted diseases. The Child Protection Centre at the Winnipeg Children's Hospital. *Ped Infect Disease J* 15: 662–667.

Harper J C (1996) Preimplantation diagnosis of inherited disease by embryo biopsy: An update of the world figures. *J Assisted Reprod Genet* 13: 90–95.

Jackson D P, Hayden J D, Quirke P (1991) Extraction of nucleic acid from fresh and archival material. In: McPherson M J, Quirke P, Taylor G R, eds. *PCR. A Practical Approach*. Oxford: IRL Press, Oxford University Press, pp. 29–50.

Kaledin A S, Slyusarenko A G, Gorodetskii S I (1982) Isolation of properties of DNA polymerases from an extreme thermophilic bacteria *Thermus aquaticus*. YT-1. *Biokhimiya* 47: 1785–1791.

Kelly K M, Womer R B, Barr F G (1996) Minimal disease detection in patients with alveolar rhabdomyosarcoma using a reverse transcriptase-polymerase chain reaction method. *Cancer* 78: 1320–1327.

Kleppe K, Ohtsuka E, Kleppe R, *et al.* (1971) Studies on polynucleotides. XCVI. Repair replications of short synthetic DNAs as catalysed by DNA polymerases. *J Mol Biol* 56: 341–361.

Lewis, R (1997) RT-PCR may ease testing of patients with thyroid cancer. *Genetic Engineering News*, March 15.

Lo Y-M D, Patel P, Wainscoat J S, *et al.* (1989) Prenatal sex determination by DNA amplification from maternal peripheral blood. *Lancet* ii: 1363–1365.

McPherson M J, Quirke P, Taylor G R (1991) In: McPherson M J, Quirke P, Taylor G R, eds. *PCR. A Practical Approach.* Oxford: IRL Press, Oxford University Press.

Markham A F (1993) The polymerase chain reaction: a tool for molecular medicine. *Brit Med J* 306(6875): 441–446.

Morris D J, Cooper R J, Barr T, Bailey A S (1996) Polymerase chain reaction for rapid diagnosis of respiratory adenovirus infection. *J Infect* 32: 113–117.

Mouritsen C L, Wittwer C T, Litwin C M, *et al.* (1996) Polymerase chain reaction detection of Lyme disease: correlation with clinical manifestations and serologic responses. *Am J Clin Pathol* 105: 647–654.

Mullis K, Faloona F (1987) Specific synthesis of DNA *in vitro* via a polymerase catalyzed chain reaction. In: Wu R, ed. *Methods in Enzymology*, Vol. 155, pp. 335–350. New York: Academic Press.

Munroe P B, Rapola J, Mitchison H M, *et al.* (1996) Prenatal diagnosis of Batten's disease. *Lancet* 347: 1014–1015.

Panet, A, Khorana G (1974) Studies of polynucleotides. The linkage of deoxyribopolynucleotide templates to cellulose and its use in their replication. *J Biol Chem* 249: 5213–5221.

Pittman K, Bradley C, Blair G E (1991) Detection of melanoma cells in peripheral blood by means of reverse transcriptase and PCR. *Lancet* 338: 1227–1229.

Quinn T C, Welsh L, Lentz A, *et al.* (1996) Diagnosis by AMPLICOR PCR of *Chlamydia trachomatis* infection in urine samples from women and men attending sexually transmitted disease clinics. *J Clin Microbiol* 34: 1401–1406.

Ross R S, Chien K R (1991) The polymerase chain reaction (PCR) and cardiovascular diagnosis. *Trends Cardiovasc Med* 1: 1–4.

Saiki R K, Scharf S, Faloona F, *et al.* (1985) Enzymatic amplification of b-globin genomic sequences and restriction site analysis for diagnosis of sickle cell anemia. *Science* 230: 1350–1354.

Saiki R K, Gelfand D H, Stoffel S, *et al.* (1988) Primer-directed enzymatic amplification of DNA with a thermostable DNA polymerase. *Science* 239: 487–494.

Schwurzer-Voit M, Proebstle T M, Sterry W (1996) Identification of lymph node metastases by use of polymerase chain reaction (PCR) in melanoma patients. *Eur J Cancer* 32A: 264–268.

Sidransky D, Von Eschenbach A, Tsai Y C, *et al.* (1991) Identification of p53 gene mutations in bladder cancers and urine samples. *Science* 252: 706–709.

Sidransky D, Tokino T, Hamilton S R, *et al.* (1992) Identification of Ras oncogene mutations in the stool of patients with curable colorectal tumours. *Science* 256: 102–105.

Stapleton M J (1996) Gene amplification for human diagnostics. *Genetic Engineering News*, 14 September.

Wujcik D (1996) Update on the diagnosis of and therapy for acute promyelocytic leukemia and chronic myelogenous leukemia. *Oncology Nursing Forum* 23: 478–487.

Yamamoto S, Pavan-Langston D, Kinoshita S, *et al.* (1996) Detecting herpesvirus DNA in uveitis using the polymerase chain reaction. *Br J Ophthamol* 80: 465–468.

6

Gene therapy for the treatment of disease

Gavin Brooks and Richard G Vile

As a direct result of the powerful techniques of genome analysis (see elsewhere in this volume), it has become possible to map, clone and sequence individual genes, mutations of which are responsible for the development of disease. Identification of such genes, and the disease-associated mutations, has raised the prospect that genetic disease may be treatable by direct correction of the underlying genetic defect – that is, at the level of the genome itself. Gene therapy was, therefore, initially conceived as a modality to treat diseases for which a (simple) genetic defect was known to be the cause. In its simplest form, gene therapy involves the delivery of an intact copy of a mutated gene into the affected cells in order to obtain long-term correction of the physiological defect caused by the original mutation. An example of such a proposed gene therapy is the treatment of cystic fibrosis (CF) by delivery of the gene for the cystic fibrosis chloride ion transporter (CFTR) protein into the airway epithelial cells of patients with CF.

However, as the number of diseases which are known to have at least some genetic component increases, so the definition of gene therapy has become much broader. Now, gene therapy is routinely evoked to encompass the use of genetic material to alleviate the symptoms of a disease, even if the therapeutic genes are not strictly 'corrective' (in the sense of restoring a function known to be mutated in the affected cells). Hence, the delivery of cytotoxic genes to kill cancer cells (rather than to correct the oncogenic mutations within them) is also accepted as gene therapy. Therefore, in its broadest terms, gene therapy represents 'an opportunity for the treatment of genetic disorders in adults and children by genetic modification of human body cells' (Report of the UK Health Minister's Gene Therapy Advisory Committee, 1995).

A further important classification is to distinguish the *heritable potential* of gene therapy. All of the gene therapy trials which are currently approved for use in human patients target those somatic cells which will live only as long as the patient. Barring inadvertent spread of the therapeutic genes to the gametes, the genetic treatment will affect only one generation and will not be able to alter the genetic make-up of any offspring of the patient. This is, therefore, known as somatic gene therapy, and its purpose is to alleviate disease in the treated individual and that individual alone.

In contrast, it also is possible to target directly the gametes (sperm and ova) in order to modify the genetic profile not of the current but of the subsequent generation of unborn 'patients'. Gene transfer at an early stage of embryonic development may also have the same effects by achieving gene transfer to both somatic and germline cells. This is germline gene therapy. The attraction of germline gene therapy for the treatment of disease is that, at least in theory, permanent genetic cures might be achieved by delivering a functional copy of a mutated gene to every cell of the resulting progeny. However, there is currently extensive apprehension about the development of germline gene therapy research programmes. The ability to alter the genetic profile of subsequent generations rightly invokes many spectres. Apart from the inability to predict the long-term sequelae of altering the germ line by delivery of exogenous genetic material at the scientific level, there are many ethical issues raised by the prospect of treating 'patients' whose consent it is impossible to obtain. In addition, although it is currently not possible to manipulate genetically traits such as 'intelligence' or 'beauty', there is a perceived fear of such technology being abused in eugenic-type breeding programmes in the future. As a result, the major ethical and regulatory bodies of gene therapy in both the US and Europe have placed a moratorium on the consideration of any germline gene therapy treatments of human patients because of 'insufficient knowledge to evaluate the risks to future generations' (Report of the UK Health Minister's Gene Therapy Advisory Committee, 1995). However, it is important that such issues be addressed at a regulatory level sooner rather than later. Non-consideration of applications for germline trials in patients will in no way prevent continued research into the direct genetic modification of the germ line, and the relevant ethical and regulatory dilemmas will simply be deferred, rather than solved, by procrastination.

Gene therapy – in search of the perfect disease

Genetically, gene therapy is well advanced for many diseases – that is, the underlying genetic defect has been identified and the corrective version of the relevant mutated gene is available for delivery and expression into target tissues. However, it is the imperfections of current *in vivo* gene delivery technologies that currently impose the most limiting restrictions upon the practical success of most proposed gene therapy protocols (Ali *et al.*, 1994; Jolly, 1994; Vile and Russell, 1994; Hodgson, 1995). Therefore, when assessing candidate diseases for suitability for gene therapy, several genetic and pragmatic considerations must be taken into account. The following checklist can be drawn up, against which a candidate disease can be compared, when considering how it relates to the 'perfect' target disease for gene therapy:

1   The pathology of the disease should be caused by a defect in just a single gene (monogenic disorders), the correction of which will restore normal physiological function to the affected cells/tissues. Hence, affected cells require only one gene to be delivered; the probability of delivering more than one gene to any given cell *in vivo* diminishes rapidly with increasing number.

2   The gene that is mutated in such a monogenic disorder should have been cloned and the mutations which cause disease should be well characterised.

3   Correction of the physiological defect caused by the mutation should be achievable by simple on/off regulation of expression of the correct version of the gene. Obtaining *temporally* regulated gene expression in target cells *in vivo* requires inclusion of regulatory elements which are still being characterised in most systems; in addition, *quantitative* regulation of exogenously introduced gene expression, relative to other endogenous genes *in vivo*, is also likely to be especially problematic.

4   Expression of the therapeutic gene should be non-toxic to normal cells so that perfectly *targeted delivery* only to the affected cell type is not required. This will permit relatively promiscuous gene delivery without widescale toxicity.

5   The target cells/tissue for gene correction should be in localised, anatomically accessible positions. Delivery of a single copy of any gene to every cell in the body is currently impossible, other than by germline or by *in utero* gene therapy. This requirement will help to overcome the problems with *efficiency* of gene delivery, which is a major limitation to gene therapy for most diseases.

6   Indeed, delivery of a single copy of a gene to every cell even in a localised body compartment is highly improbable with current technologies. Therefore, correction of the physiological defect should be achievable by delivery of the corrective gene to only a proportion of the affected target cells by means of some form of *bystander effect*.

7   Given the costs associated with the development of any new drugs for human use, and especially considering the heightened safety concerns associated with the use of genetic treatments in humans, in order to justify the many regulatory hurdles which must be traversed for the use of gene therapy, there should be no effective currently existing treatment for the disease.

Gene therapy – the real diseases

In contrast to the idealised situation described above, a wide variety of conditions have been proposed to be amenable to gene therapy, some more realistically than others (Anderson, 1992). These range from simple monogenic disorders (e.g. cystic fibrosis), which fulfil many of the criteria described above for the ideal candidate disease, through more complex monogenic and multifactorial genetic diseases (e.g. cancer), to diseases in which the underlying genetic 'defect' is introduced into the patient in the form of pathogenic genomes of bacteria or viruses (e.g. AIDS). Examples of the spectrum of diseases currently under active investigation with genetic therapies are given below; although it is not possible to describe each disease in great detail, examples are used from different classes of disease type to illustrate the potential, and pitfalls, of gene therapy.

Simple monogenic disorders

Not surprisingly, the diseases for which clinical trials are most advanced, and for which there is the most optimism for a clinical outcome, are those which conform the closest to the criteria 1–7 above. The best examples of such disorders are CF and severe combined immune deficiency (SCID).

CF is a recessive disorder caused by mutation to a single gene encoding a chloride ion transporter protein, the cystic fibrosis transporter (CFTR) (Collins, 1992). When a patient inherits two mutated copies of the CFTR gene, ion transport across epithelial surfaces is disrupted. The most life-threatening pathology of CF presents as an accumulation of thick mucus in the airways accompanied by high risks of bacterial infection. This pathology is directly attributable to a defect in chloride ion transport across the airway epithelial cells such that water is not secreted into the mucus-lined airway passages. Although CF patients also have other pathological consequences, especially in the gut and pancreas, these conditions are usually managed effectively relative to the pulmonary symptoms (Collins, 1992).

The *CFTR* gene was cloned following extensive mapping studies, and the range of mutations associated with the CF phenotype has been well documented (Collins, 1992). *In vitro* and *in vivo* studies have shown that as few as 30% of cells in sheets of affected CF epithelial cells need to express the correct version of the *CFTR* gene for normal physiological levels of chloride ion transport to be restored to the entire cell layer (Collins, 1992). Transgenic CF mouse models have also been developed which show physiologically defective chloride ion transport across their airway epithelial cells. Unfortunately, these transgenic models do not necessarily develop CF-like disease, so *therapeutic* gene therapy is difficult to demonstrate, although correction of the chloride ion transport defect has been conclusively shown (Alton *et al.*, 1993; Hyde *et al.*, 1993).

Thus, CF represents a near ideal candidate for classical gene therapy. The pathology is caused by a single-gene defect (1 above), which can be corrected in *in vitro* and *in vivo* models by expression of the correct version of the gene (2) without the need for specific temporal or quantitative regulation of its expression (3). There is no evidence that expression of the *CFTR* gene in other tissues is toxic (4), and expression of the correct gene in only a proportion of affected epithelial cells is sufficient to restore normal function to epithelial cell layers (6). The target population for gene correction is relatively accessible to gene delivery by aerosols or even direct application (5) and, although a range of conventional treatments can extend CF patients' lifespans into the mid-30s, a lack of life-long treatments for CF more than justifies the investment in gene therapy as a curative alternative (7).

Accordingly, clinical trials of delivery of the *CFTR* gene to affected airway epithelial cells have now been approved and are under way in both the UK (Caplen *et al.*, 1994) and the US (Welsh *et al.*, 1994). In the first instance, these trials are aimed at assessing safety and are unlikely to show real therapeutic effects, not least because various technical hurdles still remain to be overcome. For example, although delivery of the CFTR expression vector to the airways is physically relatively simple (using either DNA complexed with cationic liposomes or high-titre CFTR-adenoviral stocks), these vectors must penetrate the thick mucus to gain access to the epithelial cells before physiological correction can occur. It remains to be seen whether sufficient epithelial cells can be targeted in this way to generate clinical benefits to these patients.

In addition, other confounding factors associated with gene delivery make it unlikely that these early trials would be truly therapeutic. Since adenoviral vectors do not integrate into target cell chromosomes (Ali *et al.*, 1994), any cells that become successfully transduced with the gene are most likely to express it only transiently. Hence, repeated administrations of viral vector would be required for chronic correction in the patient. However, development of immunity to the virus may well prevent such repeated administrations being effective (Yang *et al.*, 1994). In addition, inflammation in the lungs of animals treated with high-titre doses of recombinant adenovirus has been reported, and one patient in a trial in the US has already developed a life-threatening inflammation reaction as a result of immune reactivity against very high-dose adenoviral stock administered into the airway passage (Yei *et al.*, 1994). Alternative trials using CFTR expression vector plasmid DNA complexed with cationic liposomes seek to avoid such inflammatory problems by excluding the use of viral vectors (Caplen *et al.*, 1994). However, what such protocols seek to gain in terms of repeatability of dosing, they lose in terms of efficiency of gene transfer. Ideally, the corrective *CFTR* gene should penetrate the mucous barrier at sufficient levels that at least some of the stem cells of the continually self-renewing epithelial cell layer become transduced. Only if stem cells can be stably transduced will the need for lifelong administrations be avoided, a dogma that holds for many different forms of gene therapy.

Initial reports on the *in vivo* correction of chloride ion transport across small, treated areas (usually of the nasal lining of CF patients) are now appearing in the literature and look cautiously hopeful (Zabner *et al.*, 1993). However, much technical work remains to be done before the inevitable compromises between efficiency and safety of gene delivery can be reconciled and trials can proceed to protocols in which genuine clinical benefits are expected.

The second simple monogenic disorder which is at the forefront of human gene therapy trials is severe combined immune deficiency (SCID). One form of SCID is caused by the absence of functional adenosine deaminase (ADA) in patients' lymphocytes. However, animal models of SCID have shown that T-cell function can be corrected by removing affected lymphocytes *ex vivo* and expressing the cloned *ADA* gene in them. Return of 'corrected' lymphocytes to the animal can then provide systemic enzyme levels that are sufficiently high for the immune system to function at normal levels (Vega, 1992). Therefore, clinical trials are now well advanced in the US in which patient lymphocytes are removed, transduced *ex vivo* with a retrovirus encoding the *ADA* gene and returned *in vivo* to act as a source of ADA enzyme (Blaese, 1990). In this instance, many of the delivery problems associated with the CF trials are overcome by the *ex vivo* isolation of the target cells, their high-level transduction by viral vectors and the potential to gain long-term, stable expression of the therapeutic gene by using a retro-viral vector that integrates into the genome (Vega, 1992).

The results of these trials (one of the first human gene therapy trials to be approved) are very encouraging, although in some respects they are still ambiguous. Since it was considered to be ethically unacceptable to withhold the existing treatment of recombinant polyethylene glycol-complexed ADA enzyme to patients treated with the genetically modi-fied lymphocytes (who now attend school and are apparently well), it has not been possible to attribute their continued immune function solely to the gene therapy rather than to the conventional treatment. Nonethe-less, lack of detectable treatment-related toxicity, detection of the intro-duced gene in circulating lymphocytes and continually elevated levels of ADA suggest that this form of gene therapy may eventually become stan-dard in the treatment of this disease.

Although ADA deficiency is one of the flagships of human clinical gene therapy, it is actually a very rare disorder. Its adoption by the gene therapy community as a prototype disease to espouse its cause is cer-tainly not driven by consideration of the existence of large numbers of desperate patients (point 7 above). Rather its amenability to the require-ments of gene therapy (points 1–6) have made it the most likely to work (Vega, 1992). Thus, it is hoped that apparent success in this disease can be used as a justification to proceed with other similar monogenic dis-orders and even with other less ideal situations. Examples of such cases include a variety of metabolic disorders whose pathology is associated with the lack of a single identified enzyme (Kay and Woo, 1994). Often restoration of 5–25% of normal *serum* enzyme activity will protect from clinical disease in conditions such as haemophilia B, caused by a lack of clotting factor IX. Therefore, the relevant gene can be delivered into ectopic tissues or *ex vivo* modified fibroblasts followed by implantation of the genetically modified cells to serve as a source of serum enzyme. Haemophiliac dogs have been 'cured' by implantation of factor IX gene-modified cells or by direct gene modification of hepatocytes with retro-viral vectors encoding the factor IX gene (Kay *et al.*, 1993), and human trials based on these results have been proposed.

In summary, there are several disorders whose properties make them conceptually very attractive as candidates for gene therapy, as defined by the criteria listed above. However, even the most theoreti-cally amenable diseases still present many technical difficulties which must be overcome before gene therapy becomes a routine tool in patient management.

Complex monogenic disorders

Treatment of certain other monogenic disorders will, however, be more complex from both the pragmatic and genetic standpoints. In these instances, simple replacement of the corrective gene either into the normal cells that produce the relevant gene product (e.g. airway epithelial cells in the case of CF) or into more easily manipulated ectopic tissues (e.g. transplanted fibroblasts for secretion of factor IX), is not likely to be sufficient to alleviate disease symptoms.

For example, some monogenic metabolic disorders will require gene modification of specific tissues that provide co-factors for enzyme activity. Hence, correction of phenylketonuria requires delivery of the phenylalanine hydroxylase enzyme specifically to liver cells because co-factors produced in hepatic cells are necessary for optimal enzyme activity. Similar requirements will be necessary for treatment of some disorders of glycogen metabolism or of the urea cycle in which normal function of therapeutic genes requires additional hepatic enzymes (Kay and Woo, 1994).

Another example of a complex monogenic disorder is the haemoglobinopathies (thalassaemias). Thalassaemias are the result of a deficiency of globin genes such that the resulting haemoglobin structures are unstable and/or defective in their normal oxygen carrying properties (Weatherall, 1985). As such, it is attractive to propose that simple delivery of the missing globin genes could be used to correct the relevant thalassaemic condition. Thus, expression of the β-globin gene in target cells could reverse β-thalassaemia (deficiency of β-globin chains). Unfortunately, synthesis of the haemoglobin tetramers involves very tight biochemical regulation, characterised by both temporal and quantitative controls on the production of several different globin species relative to each other. Therefore, simply overexpressing a particular globin molecule in the cell at any given time may only deregulate haemoglobin synthesis in a different way – for instance, by converting a β-globin thalassaemia (*relative* lack of β-globin chains) into an α-thalassaemia (*relative* lack of α-globin chains). Transcriptional control of the globin gene family is known to be highly regulated by tissue-specific enhancers and locus control regions (LCRs) (Dillon, 1993; Dillon and Grosveld, 1993), which determine the temporal switching of globin chain synthesis during development. Thus, effective gene therapy aimed at control of globin synthesis will have to incorporate such transcriptional regulation into the therapeutic constructs. Although retroviral vectors that do appear to preserve the developmental regulation pattern of globin expression have been constructed (Dzierzak *et al.*, 1988), there remains much to improve before gene therapy of thalassaemias can be confidently advanced into a clinical setting.

In summary, even though several diseases are caused by defects in just a single cloned gene (1 and 2), in many cases the central therapeutic issue focuses not upon the gene itself but on achieving the correct levels and timing of its expression (3) relative to other gene products with which the gene product must interact in the relevant biochemical pathways *in vivo*. Identification of transcriptional control elements which can *target* and *regulate* gene expression promises to be one of the most important advances in the coming years in the field of gene therapy.

Multifactorial genetic disorders

Many known diseases clearly have a genetic component but the genetic contribution is shared between several genetic loci and/or is enhanced by epigenetic factors. For example, genetic linkages have been variously reported for several psychiatric disorders, but the degree of genetic and environmental contributions remains unclear. Even when candidate genes for such diseases have been identified, as is potentially the case for Alzheimer's disease, the value of the genes for therapy remains unclear because of doubts as to the contributions of other genes and environmental influences on development of the disease (Friedmann and Jinnah, 1993).

However, an example of a disease with multiple genetic components that is widely cited as a target for gene therapy is cancer. However, if CF and ADA deficiency represent the conceptually easy end of the gene therapy spectrum, then cancer represents the other extreme (Vile and Russell, 1994). The evolution of the malignant phenotype usually involves multiple genetic lesions within the same cell (see below) (1), and it is unlikely that the nature of every one of these oncogenic mutations is known (2); most cancer patients die because their primary cancers spread throughout the body to colonise essential tissues and organs as metastases – hence, the target population for gene therapy is usually widely dispersed and often not greatly accessible (5); in addition, unlike CF or ADA deficiency, every tumour cell must, in theory, be 'corrected' to avoid the emergence of recurrent disease so that every malignant tumour cell must be targeted by the therapy (6). Therefore, it would seem that cancer would not be a natural candidate for gene therapy, because the regulated delivery of just a single gene to localised areas of affected tissues remains highly problematic (see above). Nonetheless, the majority of human gene therapy trials currently under clinical assessment are targeted towards cancer. The rationalisation of this almost certainly originates not in a common belief that cancer is particularly amenable to gene therapy, but rather in point (7) described earlier, i.e. a large patient population lacking effective, tolerable treatments.

The conversion of a normal cell into a fully transformed, malignant cell typically involves mutations in several genes of different classes (Vogelstein and Kinzler, 1993). Thus, so-called dominantly acting mutations convert proto-oncogenes into oncogenes and, within the same malignant clone, loss of function mutations abrogate the activity of tumour suppressor genes (Vile and Morris, 1992). The genetic pathway of colorectal tumorigenesis is commonly believed to involve typically about five genetic mutations (or 'hits') to both proto-oncogenes (such as *ras*) and tumour-suppressor genes (such as *p53, DCC, APC*) (Fearon and Jones, 1992). Therefore, it is far from obvious which of these genetic defects should be targeted for correction in a 'classical' gene therapy approach. It also seems improbable that, even if a single mutation could be corrected in every tumour cell, the malignant phenotype will necessarily be reversed, as the evolution of malignancy in human tumours is so multicomponent in nature.

Nonetheless, several protocols have been proposed in which a mutation that is supposedly central to the continued maintenance of the transformed phenotype is targeted within the tumour cells, with the hope that its correction may reverse the malignant phenotype or induce apoptosis. Thus, delivery of antisense constructs (Mercola and Cohen, 1995) targeted at abrogating the activity of activated oncogenes (such as *ras*) has been proposed (Georges *et al.*, 1993), as have protocols that seek to deliver a functional copy of tumour-suppressor genes that are believed to be particularly important to maintenance of the malignant phenotype (Friedmann, 1992), such as p53 (Fujiwara *et al.*, 1993). However, even if these genes are central enough to the tumorigenic process in some human cancers to be used as rational gene targets, there remains the considerable problem of delivering at least a single copy of the therapeutic gene to every tumour cell carrying the mutation (although a bystander effect, of unknown origin, has been described, which apparently leads to the killing of non-transduced tumour cells by an antisense construct to the N-*ras* gene; Georges *et al.*, 1993). Such levels of gene delivery, even to all the cells in only a localised tumour mass, let alone to systemically dispersed metastatic deposits, is currently impossible (Vile and Russell, 1994), so such strategies remain more hopeful than realistic.

As a result of these considerations, genetic therapies for cancer have been proposed which necessarily have led to the creation of a broader definition of gene therapy. These strategies (Dorudi *et al.*, 1993; Rosenberg *et al.*, 1993; Russell, 1993; Culver and Blaese, 1994;

Whartenby *et al.*, 1995) represent a fundamental departure from the gene therapies already described, wherein the aim has been to preserve affected cells by *correcting* their basic genetic defects. Instead, the majority of gene therapy protocols for cancer seek to use non-corrective genes to enhance target (tumour) cell *killing*.

Gene therapy can be used to kill tumour cells either:

1   directly, by delivery of a cytotoxic gene to the tumour cells themselves; or
2   indirectly, by the delivery of an immunomodulatory gene that activates the immune system to recognise putative tumour antigens and leads to immune-mediated cell killing.

The delivery of cytotoxic genes to tumour cells has been used essentially for the treatment of localised tumour deposits that are accessible to gene delivery but are inoperable. The most commonly used strategy involves delivering a gene encoding an enzyme that will activate a prodrug to a toxic metabolite, leading to the death of the cell expressing the gene. An example of such a system currently in clinical trials is the herpes simplex virus thymidine kinase gene (HSV*tk*) coupled with the anti-herpetic drug, ganciclovir (GCV) (Culver *et al.*, 1992). This system has the added advantage that a local bystander killing effect leads to the killing of (non-transduced) cells neighbouring the cells expressing the HSV*tk* gene as a result of transfer of toxic metabolites between juxtaposed cells (Bi *et al.*, 1993; Freeman *et al.*, 1993). Hence, in a trial at the National Institutes of Health in the United States, patients with inoperable gliomas receive retroviral vectors encoding HSV*tk* by stereotactic injection directly into the glioma followed by systemic GCV (Oldfield *et al.*, 1993). In this design of trial, the chances of success are maximised by reducing the clinical situation, as much as possible, to a classical gene therapy approach. Hence, a single gene (1) is delivered to a localised target tissue (5) in a manner requiring simple on/off regulation of expression (3), and the presence of the metabolic bystander effect means that the gene does not have to be delivered to every cell of the target cell population (6). The problem of toxicity following inadvertent delivery of the toxic gene to surrounding normal brain tissue (4) has been partly overcome in this instance by the use of retroviral vectors for gene delivery; these viruses should infect only the dividing tumour cells and cannot infect the neighbouring quiescent neural tissue (Ram *et al.*, 1993a). Similar trials using cytotoxic genes delivered to tumour masses in other anatomical locations will require other forms of targeting to ensure minimal toxicity to surrounding tissues. Although in its infancy, the technology to provide this targeting will be provided by engineering specific tropisms into the delivery vectors, for instance by the use of transcriptional targeting (Vile and Hart, 1993).

An alternative approach for cancer gene therapy is to deliver genes that enhance the immunogenicity of tumour cells, thereby augmenting the immune response against them (Rosenberg *et al.*, 1993; Tepper and Mule, 1994). Use of the immune system presents two major theoretical advantages for cancer gene therapy:

1   If it can be activated to recognise tumour-specific antigens on tumour cells, the *specificity* of the immune response should mean that systemic toxicity is reduced to a minimum, as only tumour cells expressing the antigens will be killed.
2   Once activated, immune responses have a natural *response amplification* mechanism so that only a small stimulus (low levels of gene transfer) is required to produce a large response which should, in theory, be body-wide and long-lasting.

In effect, if an immune response can be effectively activated against tumour cells, the burden of gene delivery efficiency, specificity and inadvertent toxicity should be transferred from the gene therapist onto the immune system.

There is now good evidence that at least some tumours express tumour antigens that can be recognised under certain circumstances by the immune system (Boon *et al.*, 1994). Therefore, it has been proposed that expression of various types of immunostimulatory molecules in tumour cells might enhance immune recognition, possibly by overcoming intrinsic defects in the pathways of antigen presentation by tumour cells (Pardoll, 1993). The hope is that tumour cells engineered to express such molecules, either *ex vivo* as vaccines or directly by *in vivo* gene delivery, will generate long-lasting immunity to unmodified tumour cells growing at distant sites in the body. Encouraging results have been obtained in animal studies using tumour cells modified to express cytokines [e.g. interleukin 2 (IL-2), interleukin 4 (IL-4), granulocyte–macrophage colony-stimulating factor (GM-CSF) and interferon (IFN); see Chapter 10 for further details] (Tepper and Mule, 1994), co-stimulatory molecules (e.g. members of the B7 family) (Townsend and Allison, 1993), major histocompatability complex (MHC) molecules (Browning and Bodmer, 1992; Ramarathinam *et al.*, 1994) and allogeneic antigens (Plautz *et al.*, 1993) and syngeneic tumour antigens (Hawkins *et al.*, 1993). Clinical trials in humans are under way to determine whether these results translate into clinical gains.

A modification of this approach has been to use immune cells recovered from excised tumours in adoptive transfer protocols (Rosenberg, 1991). Hence, immune cells infiltrating certain human tumours, principally melanoma, renal cell cancers and colorectal cancers, have been grown *ex vivo* to high numbers and reinfused into patients. The rationale is that the immune cells presumably have natural tumour recognition capabilities as they were originally isolated from growing tumours; when reinfused they should circulate through the body and concentrate in metastatic deposits expressing whatever antigens they are primed to recognise. Initial patient trials using non-T/non-B-cell tumour-infiltrating lymphokine-activated killer (LAK) cells in adoptive immuno-therapy (Rosenberg, 1984) were superseded by the use of a more specific T-cell population of IL-2 expanded tumour-infiltrating lymphocytes (TILs) (Rosenberg *et al.*, 1988a; Ioannides and Whiteside, 1993). Although these trials have reported only limited clinical success, TIL populations are now being used in gene therapy experiments. TILs recovered from patients will be engineered *ex vivo* to express either IL-2 or tumour necrosis factor (TNF) and will then be reinfused into the patient (Rosenberg *et al.*, 1993). Therefore, TILs are effectively being used as tumour-specific delivery vehicles to express immune activating and/or tumoricidal cytokines at high concentrations within tumour deposits. It is not possible to reach therapeutically useful concentrations of such cytokines, especially TNF, by systemic administration of recombinant proteins because of the toxicities associated with such treatments in humans. This combination of TILs and gene transfer is attractive if the TILs can genuinely localise to tumour deposits that the clinician cannot find/treat. However, the *in vivo* efficacy of TILs in most tumour types remains controversial.

Finally, gene therapy has been proposed as a means of improving the efficacy of conventional chemotherapeutic treatments. One of the commonest causes of treatment failure is the emergence of drug-resistant tumour cells (Dalton *et al.*, 1989; Endicott, 1995) that can no longer respond to levels of chemotherapy which are not unacceptably toxic to the patient. If chemotherapy doses could be increased, without the associated bone marrow toxicities, it may be that chemotherapy could be more effective against these resistant clones. Therefore, it has been proposed that transfer of the gene encoding the multidrug-resistant protein (*MDR-1*) (Endicott, 1995) into bone marrow cells may allow increased dosing with chemotherapeutic drugs (Gottesman and Pastan, 1993). Drug levels might be attainable which will now be toxic to tumour cells but will still be acceptable to the modified marrow because MDR protein actively pumps various chemotherapeutic drugs out of cells that express it.

Chemoprotective gene therapy of bone marrow cells has been effective in animal models (Sorrentino *et al.*, 1992) and may prove to be clinically beneficial in dose escalation regimens in human patients.

In summary, gene therapy for diseases that have a multifactorial genetic component, such as cancer, present many more theoretical problems than the simple monogenic disorders such as CF or ADA deficiency. For cancer in particular, the scope of gene therapy has been expanded to include the use of cytotoxic and immunomodulatory genes, as well as the more conventional corrective approaches which are more analogous to CF or ADA deficiency. However, reduction of the clinical target to as close to the CF-type situation as possible may increase the chances of success for specific clinical situations (such as the treatment of gliomas with the HSV*tk*/GCV system).

Infectious diseases

In theory, gene therapy for infectious diseases is attractive because the invading organism introduces *pathogen-specific* genetic material, which is an ideal target for genetic intervention. For example, it is possible to synthesise antisense oligonucleotides with high specificity for gene targets upon which replication of the pathogen is dependent but which should not recognise any cellular genetic material (Miller and Vile, 1994). Host target cells could then be transduced with such pathogen-protective constructs such that they become resistant to productive infection. Such approaches have been suggested as treatment for protozoan parasite infections for which drug therapy is currently inadequate (Miller and Vile, 1994).

Viral infections offer similar opportunities for specific genetic interventions. Indeed, in cancers with a known viral aetiology, the presence of viral genes upon which the evolution of the malignant phenotype depends offers more cause for optimism than in the treatment of non-viral cancers because of the presence of specific targets that are separate from cellular genes. Thus, gene therapy designed to abrogate the expression of papilloma transforming proteins E6 and E7 might be effective in the treatment of cervical cancer; similarly, hepatitis B (hepatocellular carcinoma), human T-cell lymphotropic virus types 1 and 2 (adult T-cell lymphoma/leukaemia) and Epstein–Barr virus (nasopharyngeal carcinoma and Burkitt's lymphoma) all offer virus-specific targets for gene therapy intervention in the infected target cells.

Similarly, gene therapy is becoming an increasingly attractive option for the treatment of AIDS in the continuing absence of an effective vaccine or drug treatment for HIV infection (Gilboa and Smith, 1994). HIV is a complex retrovirus whose genome expression is controlled by a series of regulatory proteins that control levels of viral protein production and the switch from latency to productive infection (Subbramanian and Cohen, 1994). One of these proteins, TAT, is an obligatory transcriptional activator of the viral promoter in the long terminal repeat (LTR). It may be possible to use the complexity of the control of genome expression against the virus to protect the principal target of HIV infection, the CD4+ T cells. For instance, T cells removed *ex vivo* can be transduced with constructs that use the HIV LTR to direct expression of a suicide gene such as the HSV*tk* gene (Brady *et al.*, 1994) (see above). When these T cells are returned *in vivo*, the absence of TAT will prevent expression of the *tk* gene. However, if the patient becomes infected with HIV, when the modified T cells become infected the wild-type virus will provide TAT *in trans* and expression of the transgene HSV*tk* will be activated. Treatment of the patient with GCV would kill the infected T cells before they could serve as a reservoir of viral production, thereby limiting the ability of HIV to infect more cells. However, such approaches would be unlikely to prevent infection and would, at best, only slow the progression of disease. Other gene therapy approaches that seek to interfere specifically with viral replication steps without killing the infected T cells have also been proposed (Dropulic and Jeang, 1994), including the transduction of CD4+ T cells with TAT-dependent HIV-specific antisense or ribozyme (Altman, 1993) constructs (Buchschacher and Panganiban, 1992). So far, *in vitro* experiments have shown promising results in that these constructs can protect tissue culture cells from infection with HIV and applications are currently being approved for trials in HIV infected patients.

Delivery systems for gene therapy

From the preceding discussions of the clinical situations in which gene therapy may have a role for the future, it is clear that the principal constraint is the ability to deliver the therapeutic gene effectively to the target cells. Vector systems must achieve gene transfer, depending upon the different clinical targets, with varying degrees of *efficiency, accuracy, stability* and *safety*. These properties will be discussed in general terms below, but for detailed reviews of the properties of individual gene delivery systems the reader is referred to other reviews (Ali *et al.*, 1994; Jolly, 1994; Vile and Russell, 1994).

Efficiency of gene transfer

Physical, non-viral methods of gene transfer have been described for the transduction of cells both *in vitro* and *in vivo*.

Generally, the most efficient means of delivering genes to cells *in vivo* has been by complexing the DNA with cationic lipid and either injecting the complex into the target tissue (e.g. tumour) (Plautz *et al.*, 1993), intravenously (Zhu *et al.*, 1993) or applying it directly onto the target tissue (Caplen *et al.*, 1994). However, these methods are usually much less efficient than using virus-mediated vectors. Viruses are natural genetic vectors and have optimised their life cycles for the carriage of genes into target cells. The use of replication-defective, recombinant viral vectors has greatly increased the possible efficiencies of gene transfer *in vivo*. To date, only recombinant retroviral vectors and adenoviral vectors have been used in clinical trials (Hodgson, 1995). Each has specific advantages and disadvantages which are reviewed elsewhere (Ali *et al.*, 1994; Jolly, 1994; Vile and Russell, 1995). With current vectors the order of decreasing efficiency of titres is adenoviral vectors > retroviral vectors > plasmid vectors.

In order to improve existing efficiencies, novel liposome formulations are being developed for plasmid-based delivery (San *et al.*, 1993; Zhu *et al.*, 1993), and improvements to viral titres have been achieved by various means (Burns *et al.*, 1993). Nonetheless, currently available vectors often lack sufficient titres for the demands of the clinical situation, and improvements in this area will be necessary, especially where the target cell population is very large (such as tumours). These considerations have led to suggestions that the only way to achieve sufficient titres for certain disorders is to develop replication-competent vectors that can initiate spreading infections within the target cell population (Russell, 1994) but which have inbuilt safety features to prevent their spread to other cell types (Vile and Russell, 1995). Currently, however, the use of such replicating vectors remains strictly a development for the future.

Accuracy of gene transfer

Ideally, the therapeutic gene should be delivered/expressed only in the target cells to prevent any treatment-related toxicities, although the importance of this requirement depends heavily upon the type of gene that is being used (Vile and Russell, 1994).

Accuracy of delivery of the vector can be achieved at several levels

(Vile, 1994; Miller and Vile, 1995). The vector can be delivered to the target area by *physical* means such as stereotactic injection into tumour deposits (HSV*tk*) (Oldfield *et al.*, 1993) or topical application onto airway epithelial cells (CF) (Zabner *et al.*, 1993). However, more sophisticated genetic means of gene targeting are required for vectors that encode potentially toxic genes and/or which are delivered systemically.

Vector-specific targeting has been used to target HSV*tk*-encoding retroviral vectors to replicating glioma cells while avoiding infection of quiescent neural tissue around the tumour (Ram *et al.*, 1993a, b). In addition, cytokine genes such as IL-2 and TNF might be targeted to tumour deposits using the intrinsic tumour-homing properties of TILs (Rosenberg *et al.*, 1993). *Surface targeting* of the delivery vehicle would be desirable, such that it only infects the appropriate cells. Incorporation of antibodies or ligands into liposomes (Ahmad *et al.*, 1993) can target physical delivery of drugs and plasmids and engineering of (retro)viral envelopes may eventually allow cell-specific infection to occur via recognition of target cell-specific molecules (such as tumour antigens) (Russell *et al.*, 1993; Salmons and Gunzburg, 1993; Valsesia-Wittmann *et al.*, 1994). To date, the most effective targeting has been achieved at the *transcriptional* level by inclusion of cell type-specific enhancer/locus control regions in the expression vector (Huber *et al.*, 1991; Vile and Hart, 1993), thereby restricting gene expression to target cell types even if delivery occurs to surrounding cells. Ultimately, the hope is that delivery vehicles will be developed which incorporate targeting at several levels, including transcriptional and surface specificity (Miller and Vile, 1995).

Stability of gene transfer

To avoid the need for repeated administrations of gene therapy treatments, stable integration of a corrective gene into at least some of the self-renewing stem cells of the target cell population would be the ideal result of a single dose. For diseases such CF or ADA deficiency, stability of expression is clearly of great importance. Plasmid DNA and retroviral vectors can integrate into host cell chromosomes (essentially at random sites), although retrovirus-mediated integration is much more efficient and precise. Adenoviral vectors, however, are maintained episomally (i.e. not integrated into the host chromosome) in infected cells and are diluted out of the target cell population when the cells divide. Therefore, the order of decreasing efficiency of generating stable gene expression is retroviral vectors > plasmid vectors > adenoviral vectors.

Safety of gene transfer

A major concern about the advent of genetic therapies for patient treatment is the uncertainty of the consequences of introducing new genetic material into patients' cells. The use of plasmid DNA alone is perceived as carrying less threat to the patient than the use of viral vectors, partly because less DNA is usually transferred and partly because viral vectors usually retain viral regulatory sequences to improve efficiency of gene transfer. In the case of retroviral vectors, these regulatory sequences may cause activation of nearby cellular proto-oncogenes following viral integration, leading to transformation of the target cell (Cornetta *et al.*, 1991; Cornetta, 1992; Gunter *et al.*, 1993), although the estimated risk of this occurring is low (Moolten and Cupples, 1992).

In addition, although *in vitro* tests for replication-competent viruses are well developed, especially for retroviral vector stocks, there is a finite chance that contaminating, potentially pathogenic replicating viruses might be co-transferred into patients along with the recombinant stocks (Miller and Buttimore, 1986). However, the amounts of such replication-competent retrovirus which must be transferred to a patient to cause disease appear to be much greater than the quantities which can routinely be detected by current *in vitro* safety tests (Donahue *et al.*, 1992; Anderson, 1993). Recombinant viral stocks are also naturally immunogenic by displaying viral antigens on their surfaces (Yang *et al.*, 1994). This may hinder the repeated use of such stocks if more than one treatment is required as immunity to the antigens would be expected after a single dose. Moreover, immune responses to even a single dose might be damaging to the patient as exemplified by a potentially life-threatening inflammatory reaction of a CF patient treated with very high-titre adenoviral stock (see above). Therefore, a ranking of currently used vectors for safety, in decreasing order, would be plasmid vectors > retroviral vectors > adenoviral vectors.

Delivery systems of the future

It is clear that, of those vectors that are currently approved for use in human trials, no single vector system is likely to possess all the desired requirements for any given situation. The rankings of these vectors for safety, efficiency and stability of gene expression do not give concordant results. Therefore, there is often likely to be conflict in the choice of the optimal vector system to use for any particular trial. For instance, where high efficiency of gene transfer should ideally be combined with long-term stable gene expression (such as in the treatment of CF), a compromise must be made between the high-titre adenoviral vectors, the stable integration of retroviral vectors and the safest option of plasmid transfer. In other situations, the dilemma as to which system to use may be less acute; for instance, transient expression of the HSV*tk* gene, or an immunomodulatory gene, in tumour cells would probably be sufficient for cytotoxic or immuno-gene therapy of cancer, and in these cases adenovirus-mediated gene transfer might, because of its optimal efficiency, prove to be the best solution.

Other viral vectors, not yet approved for clinical use, are currently in development, including herpes simplex virus, parvovirus and adeno-associated viruses (Jolly, 1994). As the number of vector systems which are sufficiently well characterised to be safely used in patients increases, so the conflicts between the different requirements of each system should be easier to resolve. It may also soon be possible to synthesise custom-designed delivery vehicles by incorporating the best features of different individual vectors into hybrid constructs that have the specific, combined properties required for the gene therapy protocol of choice (Miller and Vile, 1995).

Gene therapy in the clinic

Clinicians have generally been quick to embrace the concept of gene therapy and are already testing a variety of novel strategies that hinge on the transfer of genetic material. The targeted diseases have already been discussed in the previous sections but, for a variety of reasons, most of the clinical gene therapy protocols that have been approved to date are for the treatment of cancer patients. Most of these early trials are phase I studies performed in poor-prognosis patients with advanced-stage disease and are designed primarily to characterise the dose-limiting toxicities of the new procedures. However, as is always the case with new forms of cancer therapy, there are high hopes (perhaps too high) that these early trials will provide convincing evidence of efficacy.

For the sake of simplicity, we provide here a brief overview of the range of clinical activity using gene transfer therapies for cancer, discussing the results where interim or final reports of the clinical data have been published. The range of techniques used for these trials covers most of the issues and technology which are involved by the clinical requirements of protocols for other disease types (as discussed earlier). To illustrate this, we have categorised the various clinical strategies under seven headings as follows:

1   genetically modified cells as cancer vaccines;
2   direct delivery of foreign HLA and B7 genes to tumour cells;
3   polynucleotide vaccination against cloned tumour antigens;
4   adoptive therapy with genetically modified effector cells;
5   direct delivery of 'suicide' genes into tumour cells;
6   delivery of tumour-suppressor genes and/or antioncogenes into tumour cells;
7   transduction of haemopoietic cells with retroviral vector containing the *MDR-1* drug resistance marker gene.

For each of these categories, the rationale has already been explained in the preceding sections, and here we describe the major areas of clinical trial activity. To avoid prohibitively long reference lists that cite the primary literature involved, the reader is referred to regular updates of all of the trials referred to here which appear in the scientific journal *Human Gene Therapy*.

Genetically modified cells as cancer vaccines

Gene transfer has revitalised the field of cancer immunotherapy, and there is much interest in the use of live or killed cytokine-secreting tumour cells as anticancer vaccines. The majority of cytokine-based gene therapy trials to date have made use of IL-2-transduced cells. IL-2 mediates the expansion of T lymphocytes after initial contact with antigen and is therefore crucial for immune responsiveness and immune memory. Based on preclinical and early clinical studies with IL-2, Brenner (1992) initiated a clinical trial for the treatment of relapsed/refractory neuroblastoma in children using IL-2-transfected autologous tumour cells as a vaccine. Cellular immunity, but not humoral immunity, against the tumour was demonstrated in some patients, and there was resolution of pulmonary nodules in one patient.

GM-CSF has poor tumour growth-inhibiting effects, but vaccination with irradiated GM-CSF-transduced cells can induce long-lived systemic (T cell-mediated) anti-tumour immunity in a number of murine model systems. Based on these findings, Dranoff *et al.* (1993) have initiated a trial for the vaccination of patients with advanced melanoma using autologous (irradiated) melanoma cells transduced with the GM-CSF gene. In addition, Simons's group has started two clinical trials using irradiated autologous tumour cells transduced with the GM-CSF gene in patients with metastatic renal cell carcinoma and metastatic prostate carcinoma. Grade 1 and 2 skin toxicity was observed in the first trial.

Other trials based on similar rationales have been started using IL-4, TNF and INF-γ.

Successful and reproducible *ex vivo* gene transfer into explanted tumour cells has often proved to be difficult because of variability between tumour biopsy samples from different patients and their resistance to *ex vivo* culture. An alternative strategy has been to introduce the cytokine genes into a different cell type (cultured fibroblasts, for example), which can then be inoculated into the tumour mass or mixed with autologous tumour cells and reinjected into the patient. Thus, Sobol and co-workers are currently conducting a clinical trial for the vaccination of patients with colon carcinoma using a mixture of autologous tumour cells and fibroblasts transduced with a gene coding for IL-2 (Sobol and Royston, 1995). A second protocol for the vaccination of patients with glioblastoma using IL-2-transduced fibroblasts mixed with autologous tumour cells has also been submitted. Using a similar strategy, Lotze and Rubin (1994) have started a trial for the treatment of patients with advanced melanoma, renal cell carcinoma, breast cancer or colon cancer using autologous tumour cells mixed with IL-4-gene transduced fibroblasts. Toxic side-effects included fever, chills, diarrhoea and skin irritation, and the preliminary data show CD3+ cell infiltration, induction of vascular cell adhesion molecules and presence of tumour-specific CD4+ cells at the vaccination site in some melanoma patients.

As a simple alternative to the use of autologous tumour cells, it is possible to vaccinate patients with allogeneic tumour cell lines that have been genetically modified to secrete a cytokine. Partial MHC mismatches between the patient and the cells that are used for vaccination may then serve to enhance the recruitment of host effector cells at the site of inoculation. However, some degree of MHC haplotype matching between the vaccine and the patient is essential to ensure that host T cells reacting with tumour antigens that are present in the allogeneic cytokine-secreting cells can recognise the same antigens on the autologous tumour. Gansbacher *et al.* (1992) have initiated one clinical trial for treatment of patients with advanced HLA-A2-positive renal cell carcinoma and a second for patients with HLA-A2-positive metastatic melanoma. Patients are vaccinated with an irradiated HLA-A2-positive melanoma or renal cell carcinoma cell line engineered to secrete IL-2. Preliminary data from the first trial show stable disease in one patient. The same group has recently submitted a protocol for vaccination of patients with advanced or metastatic prostatic carcinoma using MHC class I-matched allogeneic human prostatic carcinoma cells engineered to secrete IL-2 and IFN-γ.

Similar strategies have been used by the groups of Das Gupta and Osanto. Osanto (1993) vaccinated 24 patients with HLA-1 and/or A-2 metastatic melanoma using HLA-A1/A2-matched, IL-2-transfected, irradiated melanoma cells expressing the melanoma-associated antigens MAGE-1, -2 and -3, tyrosinase and gp-100. Systemic toxicity was mild or absent, although local swelling of draining lymph nodes was observed. All patients showed inflammatory changes and cellular infiltrate of T cells, macrophages and eosinophils at the site of vaccination and in some patients at distant sites of subcutaneous metastases. Five patients showed regression of metastases.

Direct delivery of foreign HLA and B7 genes to tumour cells

Based on animal model work by Gary Nabel and co-workers (Nabel *et al.*, 1993) an immunotherapeutic approach has been developed for the treatment of malignant melanoma. In current clinical trials, a class I MHC antigen, HLA B7, is introduced into the tumour cells *in vivo* by lipofection. Liposomal DNA is administered by direct injection into the tumour tissue. Subsequent expression of allogeneic MHC antigens on tumour cells stimulates an immune response, mainly involving cytotoxic T lymphocytes, against these cells. Interestingly, an immune response is elicited not only to the foreign MHC gene but also to previously unrecognised tumour-associated antigens within the context of the self major histocompatibility complex. In Gary Nabel's preliminary trials on humans, two of the five malignant melanoma patients treated showed an immune response and one out of the five patients experienced partial remission. Since then, there have been several improvements in the liposome formulation and the HLA B7 expression plasmid and a series of follow-up trials is currently in progress.

Polynucleotide vaccination against cloned tumour antigens

Polynucleotide vaccination involves the direct intramuscular, subcutaneous or intradermal administration of a nucleic acid expression construct coding for a cloned antigen, whereupon it is taken up and expressed by muscle cells at the site of inoculation. Sustained, low-level production of the antigen by MHC-expressing cells at an ectopic location may be sufficient to elicit an immune response even where there has been anergy or tolerance to the same antigen displayed on tumour cells.

The first approved clinical trial of polynucleotide vaccination involved the construction of a personalised idiotypic vaccine for patients with low grade follicular B-cell lymphoma. Owing to the clonal origin of B-cell lymphomas, the antigen binding site of the immunoglobulin expressed on the surface membrane of the tumour cells (the idiotype) represents a unique tumour-specific antigen distinguishing the tumour cells from normal B cells. Clinical trials have shown that idiotype-specific immunity can be induced by vaccination with idiotypic immunoglobulin. However, although clinical benefit of idiotypic vaccination has clearly been demonstrated, the major limitation is the time and effort involved in the production of each patient-specific vaccine.

To prepare a personalised polynucleotide vaccine, the first step is to isolate the V genes coding for the idiotypic immunoglobulin displayed on the lymphoma cells. All rearranged V genes in the biopsy material are amplified by PCR (Chapter 5) using 'universal' primers that bind to conserved 5′ and 3′ terminal sequences (framework one and J region). The amplified V-gene sequences are then subcloned and 10 are sequenced. Because of the abundance of lymphoma cells in the biopsy material, the lymphoma V-gene sequences can be identified by virtue of their repetition. The idiotypic VH and VL are then assembled into a scFv by a two-stage PCR and the PCR product is cloned into a mammalian cell expression vector.

The clinical trial is a phase I dose escalation (from 100 to 500 µg of plasmid DNA) in patients with advanced, refractory follicular lymphoma. So far, three patients have been vaccinated without obvious toxicity and anti-idiotypic antibodies have been detected in two of the vaccinated patients.

Adoptive therapy with genetically modified effector cells

Several trials have explored the adoptive transfer of genetically altered lymphocytes, which home to the tumour, in order to deliver a cytokine at the tumour site and to enhance the cytolytic activity of the lymphocytes. TILs can be extracted from tumour biopsies and activated/expanded by growing them in the presence of IL-2. In the first trials by Rosenberg *et al.* (1988b), reinfusion of TILs that were cultured for several weeks in IL-2 gave a 38% response rate in patients with advanced melanoma with evidence of tumour-homing by the reinfused TILs. However, tumour regression was dependent on simultaneous treatment with recombinant IL-2, and there were very few complete responses.

To enhance the benefit of adoptive immunotherapy, Rosenberg *et al.* (1988b) therefore chose to explore the use of genetically modified TILs. A first clinical trial was conducted to determine whether genetically manipulated TILs could be safely injected, and would not persist in patients. TILs were transduced with the *Neo*[R] gene using retroviral transfection, and *in vitro* assays showed no alteration of phenotype or function compared with non-transduced cells. No safety problems or toxicities were observed in 10 patients injected with the transduced TILs, and there was no observable toxicity that could be attributed to the *Neo*[R] gene. Using PCR to detect the *Neo*[R] gene, the gene-modified TILs could be detected in tumour deposits for up to 69 days and in peripheral blood for up to 189 days.

A clinical trial is currently ongoing in which patients with advanced cancer are treated with TILs that have been transduced with the gene coding for TNF-α. The idea is that the gene-modified TILs will home efficiently to the tumour deposits, resulting in a high local concentration of TNF, and thereby circumvent the toxic side-effects caused by the high doses of TNF that are necessary for an anti-tumour effect. Preliminary results of the trial show no side-effects of the treatment, and one patient who has received TNF-TILs and IL-2 has shown regression of tumour.

Other trials using TILs transduced with the *Neo*[R] gene are currently being conducted by Favrot *et al.* (1992) (TIL-*Neo*[R] in combination with rIL-2 for the treatment of patients with metastatic melanoma or renal carcinoma), Lotze *et al.* (1992) (TIL-*Neo*[R] in combination with IL-2 and IL-4 for the treatment of melanoma) and Economou *et al.* (1992) [combinations of *Neo*[R]-transduced TILs or peripheral blood lymphocytes (bulk, CD8[+] or CD4[+]) alone or in combination with IL-2 and IFN-α for the treatment of metastatic melanoma and metastatic renal cell carcinoma].

Direct delivery of 'suicide' genes into tumour cells

In less than a decade since the delivery of suicide genes to kill cancer cells was proposed, a whole range of clinical trials in humans have begun.

The protocol by Culver *et al.* (1994) uses a replication-deficient retroviral vector to transduce tumour cells comprising the highly malignant brain cancer glioblastoma multiforme. In order to obtain effective viral titres, retrovirus-producing mouse fibroblasts (rather than the retro-virus itself) are implanted into the target tumour tissue after patients have undergone surgery to remove the bulk of the brain tumour. Patients must all have failed standard therapy and have recurrent primary brain tumours with an expected survival of weeks to a few months. The treatment procedure involves (day 0) surgical debulking of the brain tumour followed by infiltration of the cavity with HSV*tk* vector-producing cells. On day 7, the patient undergoes a brain scan and, on day 8, is administered a further 5–10 ml of vector-producing cells via an Ommaya reservoir. On day 15, GCV treatment is initiated and continues for a further 14 days. Repeat administration of vector-producing cells is carried out on day 35, followed by another cycle of GCV treatment 14 days later (days 42–56). This completes the initial treatment course. Early results recently published show lack of toxicity and some tumour shrinkages but very low levels of transduction of cells in the human tumours.

In addition to therapy of central nervous system (CNS) malignancies, the HSV*tk* retroviral system has also been used for the treatment of melanomas, myelomas and ovarian cancers. The approach to treatment of ovarian cancer by Freeman *et al.* (1995) also comprises an immunological element. Instead of using mouse fibroblasts, Freeman uses a human ovarian carcinoma cell line, PA1, transduced with an HSV*tk*-containing retroviral vector. Experiments in immunodeficient mice have shown that the effects of GCV alone are not sufficient for tumour rejection. Systemic immunity is an additional requirement. Freeman's method does not involve transfer of the modified retrovirions to the patient's tumour cells. Rather, the PA1 cell line is transduced with the vector produced in a separate packaging cell line. In effect, therefore, Freeman introduces into the patient a foreign ovarian *tk*-positive tumour cell line which, upon destruction with GCV, releases tumour antigens that trigger an immune response within the patient. By virtue of the fact that the implanted cell line may share tumour antigens with the patient's tumour cells, this immune response should be effective against both the foreign cell antigens and against the patient's own tumour cells. This approach does not therefore involve *in vivo* gene transfer.

Delivery of tumour-suppressor genes and/or antioncogenes into tumour cells

Mutations in the *p53* gene contribute to the development of up to 50% of all human cancers. A clinical protocol submitted by Dr Gary Clayman of the University of Texas proposes to conduct *p53* gene transfer experiments on 21 adult patients suffering from head and neck squamous cell carcinoma. Gene transfer is achieved by intratumoral injection of the replication-defective type 5 adenovirus vector, Ad5CMV-p53, which contains the normal human p53 tumour-suppressor gene. The E1 region of Ad5CMV-p53 has been replaced with a p53 expression cassette containing the human cytomegalovirus (CMV) promoter. This and other similar trials have recently received approval in the United States.

Transduction of haemopoietic cells with retroviral vector containing the *MDR-1* drug resistance gene

Autologous bone marrow transplantation (AuBMT) is widely used to supplement intensive chemotherapy of cancers. Unfortunately, many patients relapse following AuBMT, and in those patients the marrow graft is too fragile to endure further intensive post-transplant chemotherapy. The rationale of transferring *MDR-1* gene into patients' haemopoietic stem cells is to try to make those stem cells and their offspring more resistant to the toxic effects of chemotherapy. This should allow the patients to receive higher doses of chemotherapeutic agents, which should theoretically increase the likelihood that their tumour cells can be ablated.

Five clinical trials carried out by four different groups are under way, but no results have yet been published. The trials follow a similar clinical strategy and are focused on only a few types of solid malignancy, such as breast cancer, ovarian cancer, brain tumour and lymphoma. Briefly, both bone marrow and peripheral blood cells are collected from patients; one-third to one-half of the cells are CD34 selected to reduce further the risk of tumour cell contamination in bone marrow/peripheral blood; the CD34-positive fraction is then transfected with a retroviral vector bearing the *MDR-1* gene and reinfused together with untransduced cells to the patients after preparative chemotherapy. Intensive post-transplant salvage chemotherapy will be administered at the time of relapse, coupled with an attempt to find evidence of myeloprotection conferred by the *MDR-1* gene.

Gene therapy – an extension of rational drug design

The pharmaceutical and biotechnology industries currently devote many resources to the screening of compounds for therapeutic activity, as well as to the design of small molecules aimed at the blocking, inhibition or selective binding to proteins known to be important in different disease processes. In many ways, gene therapy represents an extension of rational drug design, where the drug is a piece of nucleic acid (the gene). The relative advantages and disadvantages of small molecules over gene therapies remain to be demonstrated as gene therapies are only just beginning to be tested in clinical trials where true efficacy might be expected. Theoretically, the approach of screening and/or design of small molecules allows many more random, as well as specific, candidates to be tested, and combinatorial chemistry offers huge potential in this respect. In contrast, routine screening for the effects of different genes is currently much less convenient, although a rational choice of appropriate candidate genes can be directly made from the extensive knowledge of the molecular genetics of most target diseases.

Whatever the theoretical advantages/disadvantages of gene therapy over other pharmaceutical approaches may be, several common hurdles remain. Of these, a major obstacle is the identification of a delivery system that can deposit sufficiently high concentrations of the therapeutic product at the relevant site, without inducing significant toxicity to other cells and tissues. It is the combination of gene therapy, along with the biological vectoring systems proposed to deliver it, which may give gene therapy a target cell specificity that is difficult to achieve with conventional single target small drugs.

Over the past 5 years the promise attributed to the advent of gene therapy into the clinic has far surpassed its returns. There are now in excess of 200 clinical trials in progress worldwide using gene transfer therapies, but the results of these early phase I trials are often viewed as disappointing. However, this perception is misleading since phase I trials are not designed to return efficacy data and, in fact, no long-term adverse effects have been reported from any trials using transfer of genes into patients making this aspect of the gene therapy trials actually extremely successful. Nonetheless, to avoid the promotion of ineffective new therapies, or, equally, to avoid the rejection of potentially useful new advances in the clinic, it is important to delineate the measures by which any new therapy/drug is considered to be a success. In general, the criteria which are useful are that the new therapy should provide any, or all, of the following:

1   better survival rates;
2   better quality of life for the same survival rates;
3   combination with existing modalities to give either better quality of life and/or survival rates.

One of the major hopes for the use of gene therapy is that it will provide a much improved therapeutic index over the currently used alternative treatments. Hence, in the short term, gene therapy's potential to improve the quality of life of patients, while not reducing their survival, must be the primary goal, and expectations for more dramatic results in the first instance will be both unrealistic and damaging to the eventual development of the field. Undoubtedly, there must still be significant advances in various aspects of this discipline – notably in the development of delivery systems of high efficiency, accuracy and safety – but as molecular technology improves it is hoped that more spectacular achievements will be possible, although these advances will require time, investment and patience.

Gene therapy – the future

When contemplating the 'perfect' disease for which intervention by gene therapy stands the greatest chance of success, several criteria can be proposed by which such a disease should be selected. This disease should be a simple monogenic disorder for which the gene has been cloned and which requires simple high level expression for correction; also, the corrective gene should not be toxic to other cells if inadvertently expressed in them, but the affected cells should be accessible to gene delivery in a localised group and correction of the target cells should be achievable even if only a fraction of the cells actually receive the gene. Finally, it would only be worthwhile developing gene therapy if the disease has no simple, safe and cheap treatment already.

In reality, gene therapy, in some form or other, has been proposed for a range of different diseases, although many do not conform at all closely to the above checklist. In the case of the most idealised real disease for which gene therapy has apparently been most successful, ADA deficiency, there are actually fewer patients who suffer from the disease than researchers working on it. In contrast, cancer, the disease that least fits these criteria, is the one for which the majority of human trials currently exists, principally because many cancers have such poor prognoses that any novel therapeutic approach can be justified on the grounds of patient desperation.

Gene therapy for cancer and infectious diseases, such as AIDS, has also led to a general broadening of the definition of gene therapy away from the original concept of the use of genes to correct genetic defects within target cells. However, the unrealistic expansion of the remit of gene therapy for treatment of disease also poses some serious threats to the credibility of the field for the future. Inflated claims regarding its clinical potential, in part as a justification to obtain dwindling research funding, will raise expectations so high that even moderate clinical success in a few limited disease situations will be unable to fulfil the overhyped promise associated with gene therapy. It is important to define realistic and obtainable goals that gene therapy might actually be able to achieve. These goals will only be sensible if there is a clear knowledge of the capabilities, and limitations, of the gene delivery vectors which are currently available, and these should be well understood.

We are currently in an exciting phase where the results of the first human clinical trials of gene therapy are beginning to be reported. The first priority is to ensure that the treatments administered to patients are safe and do not cause adverse reactions. It is unlikely that these early trials will show therapeutic effects, partly because of their inherent design and partly because it is generally end-stage patients who have been recruited. Provided no unforeseen toxicities are reported, the next decade should see gene therapies being administered to patients at earlier stages of disease, in circumstances where they may begin to have therapeutic effects. Eventually, it is to be hoped that, in certain well-designed clinical situations, gene therapy may emerge as an effective adjuvant therapy for pre-existing treatment modalities and even, in some cases, as the treatment of choice in diseases as diverse as CF, cancer and AIDS.

References

Ahmad I, Longenecker M, Samuel J, Allen T M (1993) Antibody targeted delivery of doxorubicin entrapped in sterically stabilized liposomes can eradicate lung cancer in mice. *Cancer Res* 53: 1484–1488.

Ali M, Lemoine N, Ring C J A (1994) The use of DNA viruses as vectors for gene therapy. *Gene Ther* 1: 367–384.

Altman S (1993) RNA enzyme-directed gene therapy. *Proc Natl Acad Sci USA* 90: 10898–10900.

Alton E W F W, Middleton P G, Caplen N J, *et al.* (1993) Non-invasive liposome-mediated gene delivery can correct the ion transport defect in cystic fibrosis mutant mice. *Nature Genet* 5: 135–142.

Anderson W F (1992) Human gene therapy *Science* 256: 808–813.

Anderson W F (1993) What about those monkeys that got T-cell lymphoma? *Hum Gene Ther* 4: 1–2.

Bi W L, Parysek L M, Warnick R., Stambrook P J (1993) *In vitro* evidence that metabolic cooperation is responsible for the bystander effect observed with HSV tk retroviral gene therapy. *Hum Gene Ther* 4: 725–731.

Blaese R M (1990) Clinical protocol: treatment of severe combined immune deficiency (SCID) due to adenosine deaminase deficiency with autologous lymphocytes transduced with a human ADA gene. *Hum Gene Ther* 1: 327–362.

Boon T, Cerottini J C, Van den Eynde B, *et al.* (1994) Tumor antigens recognised by T lymphocytes. *Annu Rev Immunol* 12: 337–365.

Brady H J M, Miles C G, Pennington D J, Dzierzak E A (1994) Specific ablation of human immunodeficiency virus Tat-expressing cells by conditionally toxic retroviruses. *Proc Natl Acad Sci USA* 91: 365–369.

Brenner M K (1992) Phase I study of cytokine-gene modified autologous neuroblastoma cells for treatment of relapsed/refractory neuroblastoma. *Hum Gene Ther* 3: 665–676.

Browning M J, Bodmer W F (1992) MHC antigens and cancer: implications for T-cell surveillance. *Curr Opin Immunol* 4: 613–618.

Buchschacher G L, Panganiban A T (1992) Human immunodeficiency virus vectors for inducible expression of foreign genes. *J Virol* 66: 2731–2739.

Burns J C , Friedmann T , Driever W, *et al.* (1993) Vesicular stomatitis virus G glycoprotein pseudotyped retroviral vectors: concentration to very high titer and efficient gene transfer into mammalian and nonmammalian cells. *Proc Natl Acad Sci USA* 90: 8033–8037.

Caplen N J, Gao X, Hayes P, *et al.* (1994) Gene therapy for cystic fibrosis in humans by liposome-mediated DNA transfer: the production of resources and the regulatory process. *Gene Ther* 1: 139–147.

Collins F S (1992) Cystic fibrosis: molecular biology and therapeutic implications. *Science* 256: 774–779.

Cornetta K (1992) Safety aspects of gene therapy. *Br J Haematol* 80: 421–426.

Cornetta K, Morgan R A, Anderson W F (1991) Safety issues related to retroviral-mediated gene transfer in humans. *Hum Gene Ther* 2: 5–14.

Culver K W, Blaese R M (1994) Gene therapy for cancer. *Trends Genet* 10: 174–178.

Culver K W, Ram Z, Wallbridge S, *et al.* (1992) *In vivo* gene transfer with retroviral vector-producer cells for treatment of experimental brain tumors. *Science* 256: 1550–1552.

Culver K W, Link C J, Carlstrom T, *et al.* (1994) Gene therapy for the treatment of malignant brain tumours with *in vivo* tumour transduction with the herpes simplex thymidine kinase gene/ganciclovir system. *Hum Gene Ther* 5: 343–379.

Dalton W S, Grogan T M, Meltzer P S, *et al.* (1989) Drug resistance of multiple myeloma and non-Hodgkin's lymphoma: detection of P-glycoprotein and potential circumvention by addition of verapamil to chemotherapy. *J Clin Oncol* 7: 415–424.

Dillon N (1993) Regulating gene expression in gene therapy. *Trends Biotechnol* 11: 167–173.

Dillon N, Grosveld F (1993) Transcriptional regulation of multigene loci: multilevel control. *Trends Genet* 9: 134–137.

Donahue R E, Kessler S W, Bodine D, *et al.* (1992) Helper virus induced T cell lymphoma in non human primates after retroviral mediated gene transfer. *J Exp Med* 176: 1125–1135.

Dorudi S, Northover J A, Vile R G (1993) Gene transfer therapy in cancer. *Br J Surg* 80: 566–572.

Dranoff G, Jaffee E, Lazenby A, *et al*. (1993) Vaccination with irradiated tumor cells engineered to secrete murine granulocyte–macrophage colony-stimulating factor stimulates potent, specific and long lasting anti-tumor immunity. *Proc Natl Acad Sci USA* 90: 3539–3543.

Dropulic B, Jeang K T (1994) Gene therapy for human immunodeficiency virus infection: genetic antiviral strategies and targets for intervention. *Hum Gene Ther* 5: 927–939.

Dzierzak E A, Papayannopoulou T, Mulligan R C (1988) Lineage-specific expression of a human β-globin gene in murine bone marrow transplant recipients reconstituted with retrovirus-transduced stem cells. *Nature* 331: 35–41.

Economou J S, Belldegrun A, Figlin R A, *et al*. (1992) The treatment of patients with metastatic melanoma and renal cell cancer using *in vitro* expanded and genetically-engineered (neomycin phosphotransferase) bulk, CD8(+) and/or CD4(+) tumor infiltrating lymphocytes and bulk, CD8(+) and/or CD4(+) peripheral blood leukocytes in combination with recombinant interleukin-2 alone, or with recombinant interleukin-2 and recombinant alpha interferon. *Hum Gene Ther* 3: 411–430.

Endicott J A (1995) The molecular basis of resistance of cancer cells to chemotherapy. In: Vile R G, ed. *Cancer Metastasis: From Mechanisms to Therapies*. Chichester: John Wiley and Sons, 123–144.

Favrot M C, Merrouche Y, Negrier S, *et al*. (1992) Treatment of patients with advanced cancer using tumor infiltrating lymphocytes transduced with the gene of resistance to neomycin. *Hum Gene Ther* 3: 533–542.

Fearon E R, Jones P A (1992) Progressing toward a molecular description of colorectal cancer development. *FASEB J* 6: 2783–2790.

Freeman S M, Abboud C N, Whartenby K A, *et al*. (1993) The 'bystander effect': tumor regression when a fraction of the tumor mass is genetically modified. *Cancer Res* 53: 5274–5283.

Freeman S M, McCune C, Robinson W, *et al*. (1995) The treament of ovarian cancer with a gene modified cancer vaccine: a phase I study. *Hum Gene Ther* 6: 927–939.

Friedmann T (1992) Gene therapy of cancer through restoration of tumor-suppressor functions. *Cancer* (Suppl.) 70 1810–1817.

Friedmann T, Jinnah H A (1993) Gene therapy for disorders of the nervous system. *Trends Biotechnol* 11: 192–197.

Fujiwara T, Grimm E A, Mukhopadhyay, T *et al*. (1993) A retroviral wild-type p53 expression vector penetrates human lung cancer spheroids and inhibits growth by inducing apoptosis. *Cancer Res* 53: 4129–4133.

Gansbacher B, Houghton A, Livingston P, *et al*. (1992) A pilot study of immunization with HLA-A2 matched allogeneic melanoma cells that secrete interleukin-2 in patients with metastatic melanoma. *Hum Gene Ther* 3: 677–690.

Georges R N, Mukhopadhyay T, Zhang Y, *et al* (1993) Prevention of orthotopic human lung cancer growth by intratracheal instillation of a retroviral antisense K-ras construct. *Cancer Res* 53: 1743–1746.

Gilboa E, Smith C (1994) Gene therapy for infectious diseases: the AIDS model. *Trends Genet* 10: 109–114.

Gottesman M M, Pastan I (1993) Biochemistry of multidrug resistance mediated by the multidrug transporter. *Annu Rev Biochem* 62: 385–427.

Gunter K C, Khan A S, Noguchi P D (1993) The safety of retroviral vectors. *Hum Gene Ther* 4: 643–645.

Hawkins R E, Winter G, Hamblin T J, *et al.* (1993) A genetic approach to idiotypic vaccination. *J Immunother* 14: 273–278.

Hodgson C (1995) The vector void in gene therapy. *Biotechnology* 13: 222–225.

Huber B E, Richards C A, Krenitsky T A (1991) Retroviral-mediated gene therapy for the treatment of hepatocellular carcinoma: an innovative approach for cancer therapy. *Proc Natl Acad Sci USA* 88: 8039–8043.

Hyde S C, Gill D R, Higgins C F, *et al.* (1993) Correction of the ion transport defect in cystic fibrosis transgenic mice by gene therapy. *Nature* 362: 250–255.

Ioannides C G, Whiteside T L (1993) T cell recognition of human tumors: implications for molecular immunotherapy of cancer. *Clin Immunol Immunopathol* 66: 91–106.

Jolly D (1994) Viral vector systems for gene therapy. *Cancer Gene Ther* 1: 51–64.

Kay M A, Woo, S L C (1994) Gene therapy for metabolic disorders. *Trends Genet* 10: 253–257.

Kay M A, Rothenberg S, Landen C N, *et al.* (1993) *In vivo* gene therapy of hemophilia B: sustained partial correction in factor IX-deficient dogs. *Science* 262: 117–119.

Lotze M T, Rubin J T (1994) Gene therapy of cancer: a pilot study of IL-4-gene-modified fibroblasts admixed with autologous tumor to elicit an immune response. *Hum Gene Ther* 5: 41–55.

Lotze M T, Rubin J T, Edington H D, *et al.* (1992) The treatment of patients with melanoma using interleukin-2, interleukin-4 and tumor infiltrating lymphocytes. *Hum Gene Ther* 3: 167–177.

Mercola D, Cohen, J S (1995) Antisense approaches to cancer gene therapy. *Cancer Gene Ther* 2: 47–59.

Miller A D, Buttimore C (1986) Redesign of retrovirus packaging cell line to avoid recombination leading to helper virus formation. *Mol Cell Biol* 6: 2895–2902.

Miller N, Vile R G (1994) Gene transfer and antisense nucleic acid techniques. *Parasitol Today* 10: 92–97.

Miller N, Vile R G (1995) Targeted vectors for gene therapy. *FASEB J* 9: 190–199.

Moolten F L, Cupples L A (1992) A model for predicting the risk of cancer consequent to retroviral gene therapy. *Hum Gene Ther* 3: 479–486.

Nabel G J, Nabel E G, Yang Z Y, *et al.* (1993) Direct gene transfer with DNA-liposome complexes in melanoma: expression, biologic activity and lack of toxicity in humans. *Proc Natl Acad Sci USA* 90: 11307–11311.

Oldfield E H, Ram Z, Culver K W, *et al.* (1993) Clinical protocol: gene therapy for the treatment of brain tumors using intra-tumoral transduction with the thymidine kinase gene and intravenous ganciclovir. *Hum Gene Ther* 4: 39–69.

Osanto S (1993) Immunization with interleukin-2 transfected melanoma cells. A phase I–II study in patients with metastatic melanoma. *Hum Gene Ther* 4: 323–330.

Pardoll D M (1993) Cancer vaccines. *Immunol Today* 14: 310–316.

Plautz G E, Yang Z-Y, Wu B-Y, *et al.* (1993) Immunotherapy of malignancy by *in vivo* gene transfer into tumors. *Proc Natl Acad Sci USA* 90: 4645–4649.

Ram Z, Culver K W, Walbridge S, *et al.* (1993a) Toxicity studies of retroviral-mediated gene transfer for the treatment of brain tumors. *J Neurosurg* 79: 400–407.

Ram Z, Culver K W, Walbridge S, *et al.* (1993b) *In situ* retroviral mediated gene transfer for the treatment of brain tumours in rats. *Cancer Res* 53: 83–88.

Ramarathinam L, Castle M, Wu Y, Liu Y (1994) T cell co-stimulation by B7/BB1 induces CD8 T cell-dependent tumor rejection: an important role of B7/BB1 in the induction, recruitment, and effector function of antitumor T cells. *J Exp Med* 179: 1205–1214.

Report of the United Kingdom Health Minister's Gene Therapy Advisory Committee (1995) Guidance on making proposals to conduct gene therapy research on human subjects. *Hum Gene Ther* 6: 335–346.

Rosenberg S A (1984) Immunotherapy of cancer by systemic administration of lymphoid cells plus interleukin-2. *J Biol Resp Modifiers* 3: 501–511.

Rosenberg S A (1991) Immunotherapy and gene therapy of cancer. *Cancer Res* 51 (Suppl.), 5074s–5079s.

Rosenberg S A, Packard B S, Read E J, *et al.* (1988a) Use of tumor-infiltrating lymphocytes and interleukin-2 in the immuno-therapy of patients with metastatic melanoma. A preliminary report. *N Engl J Med* 319: 1676–1680.

Rosenberg S A, Packard B S, Aebersold P M, *et al.* (1988b) Use of tumor-infiltrating lymphocytes and interleukin-2 in the immunotherapy of patients with metastatic melanoma, special report. *N Engl J Med* 319: 1676–1680.

Rosenberg S A, French Anderson W, Blaese M, *et al.* (1993) The development of gene therapy for the treatment of cancer. *Ann Surg* 218: 455–464.

Russell S J (1993) Gene therapy for cancer. *Cancer J* 6: 21–25.

Russell S J (1994) Replicating vectors for cancer therapy: a question of strategy. *Semin Cancer Biol* 5: 437–443.

Russell S J, Hawkins R E, Winter G (1993) Retroviral vectors displaying functional antibody fragments. *Nucleic Acids Res* 21: 1081–1085.

Salmons B, Gunzburg W H (1993) Targeting of retroviral vectors for gene therapy. *Hum Gene Ther* 4: 129–141.

San H, Yang Z-Y, Pompili V J, *et al.* (1993) Safety and short-term toxicity of a novel cationic lipid formulation for human gene therapy. *Hum Gene Ther* 4: 781–788.

Sobol R E, Royston I (1995) Injection of colon carcinoma patients with autologous irradiated tumor cells and fibroblasts genetically modified to secrete interleukin-2 (IL-2): a phase I study. *Hum Gene Ther* 6: 195–204.

Sorrentino B P, Brandt S J, Bodine D, *et al.* (1992) Selection of drug resistant bone marrow cells in vivo after retroviral transfer of human MDR1. *Science* 257: 99–103.

Subbramanian R, Cohen E A (1994) Molecular biology of the human immunodeficiency virus accessory proteins *J Virol* 68: 6831–6835.

Tepper R I, Mule J J (1994) Experimental and clinical studies of cytokine gene-modified tumor cells. *Hum Gene Ther* 5: 153–164.

Townsend S E, Allison J P (1993) Tumour rejection after direct co-stimulation of CD8+ T cells by B7-transfected melanoma cells. *Science* 259: 368–370.

Valsesia-Wittmann S, Drynda A, Deleage G, *et al.* (1994) Modifications in the binding domain of avian retrovirus envelope protein to redirect the host range of retroviral vectors. *J Virol* 68: 4609–4619.

Vega M A (1992) Adenosine deaminase deficiency: a model system for human somatic cell gene correction therapy. *Biochim Biophys Acta* 1138: 253–260.

Vile R G (1994) Tumour specific gene expression. *Semin Cancer Biol* 5: 429–436.

Vile R G, Hart I R (1993) Use of tissue-specific expression of the Herpes simplex virus thymidine kinase gene to inhibit growth of established murine melanomas following direct intratumoral injection of DNA. *Cancer Res* 53: 3860–3864.

Vile R G, Morris A G (1992) The multiple molecular mechanisms of cancer: in search of unification. In: Vile, R G, ed. *Introduction to the Molecular Genetics of Cancer*. Chichester: John Wiley and Sons, 1–32.

Vile R G, Russell S J (1994) Gene transfer technologies for the gene therapy of cancer. *Gene Ther* 1: 88–98.

Vile R G, Russell S J (1995) Retroviruses as vectors. *Br Med Bull* 51: 12–30.

Vogelstein B, Kinzler K W (1993) The multistep nature of cancer. *Trends Genet* 9: 138–141.

Weatherall D J (1985) *The New Genetics and Clinical Practice*, 2nd edn. Oxford: Oxford Medical Publications, 71–86.

Welsh M J, Smith A E, Zabner J, *et al.* (1994) Clinical protocol: cystic fibrosis gene therapy using an adenovirus vector: *in vivo* safety and efficacy in nasal epithelium. *Hum Gene Ther* 5: 209–219.

Whartenby K A, Abboud C N, Marrogi A J, *et al.* (1995) The biology of cancer gene therapy. *Lab Invest* 72: 131–145.

Yang Y, Nunes F A, Berencsi K, *et al.* (1994) Cellular immunity to viral antigens limits E1-deleted adenoviruses for gene therapy. *Proc Natl Acad Sci USA* 91: 4407–4411.

Yei S, Mittereder N, Wer S, *et al.* (1994) *In vivo* evaluation of the safety of adenovirus-mediated transfer of the human cystic fibrosis transmembrane conductance regulator cDNA to the lung *Hum Gene Ther* 5: 731–744.

Zabner J, Couture L A, Gregory R J, *et al.* (1993) Adenovirus-mediated gene transfer transiently corrects the chloride transport defect in nasal epithelia of patients with cystic fibrosis. *Cell* 75: 1–20.

Zhu N, Liggitt,D, Liu Y, Debs, R (1993) Systemic gene expression after intravenous DNA delivery into adult mice. *Science* 261: 209–211.

7

Potential of antisense oligonucleotides as drugs

Ian Gibson

The development of oligonucleotides (also termed oligodeoxynucleotides) as therapeutic agents (Stull and Szoka, 1995), utilising a new rational approach to drug development, stems from the belief that they will intervene in a sequence-specific manner during the synthesis of a key protein (Stephenson and Zamecnik, 1978; Zamecnik and Stephenson, 1978). This may involve them binding to the messenger RNA transcribed from the gene or, indeed, by directly binding to the target gene itself. This approach can be applied to the inhibition of the synthesis of a particular host protein or to a protein required for the replication of an invading bacterium or virus. While going through various 'boom and bust' periods, this technology is now considered seriously for its potential to promote wound healing and for the treatment of hypertension, autoimmune and cardiovascular diseases, viral and other infections, e.g. HIV, and for many cancers where the genetic basis is understood (Wickstrom, 1991).

This chapter will describe the successes of the approach, the problems, the clinical trials and how the science of antisense technology is being developed by many venture capital companies. First a little history and technical explanation of the approach is required.

The science of antisense

In 1953, the discovery of the double-stranded model of DNA opened up the world of molecular biology, which eventually led to an understanding of how the amino acid sequence within a polypeptide chain was determined from information inherent in the DNA sequence of the nucleotides that make up any gene. The prediction and discovery of a small RNA molecule – transfer RNA – provided the link for the language of nucleotides to be translated into the language of amino acids. A particular transfer RNA molecule carried the *relevant* amino acid to the ribosomal machinery, where the polypeptide chain was sequentially synthesised (see Chapter 1). However, it was the process of base pair complementarity that ensured that the sequence of nucleotides in the transfer RNA formed a double-stranded RNA link with a messenger RNA sequence, which in its turn was produced by the DNA sequence. A trinucleotide sequence in the messenger RNA formed this link with the complementary sequence in the transfer RNA by base pairing rules.

It was this knowledge that suggested the possibility of intervening in the process of synthesis of a protein at the level of nucleotide sequence by forming an 'artificial' nucleotide double-stranded structure. As Figure 7.1 shows, there is the possibility of preventing the synthesis of a protein by forming an mRNA link with a small complementary DNA or oligomer or RNA sequence produced from a plasmid or vector that produces the complementary RNA. This is the basis of the antisense approach, which has a simple philosophy but in theory could result in a highly specific effect on one sequence only and, indeed, might become sophisticated enough to distinguish between two nucleotide sequences differing in one base only – a situation that features in several important diseases in which a single base mutation occurs within a gene.

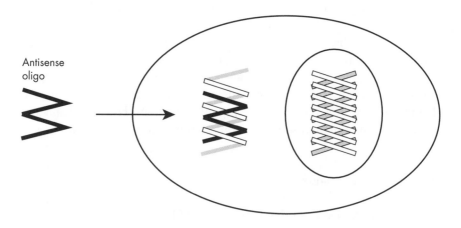

Antisense
oligo

Figure 7.1   Antisense oligodeoxynucleotide binds to complementary sequence in mRNA preventing translation. Reproduced with permission from Cohen J, ed. (1989) *Oligodeoxynucleotides. Antisense Inhibitors of Gene Expression.* Macmillan Press.

First, however, before looking at the successes and failures of the approach I shall look at the requirements for a drug over and above this potential for high genetic specificity.

Requirements of a genetic drug

Firstly there is a requirement to be able to synthesise large quantities of the drug. The cost of manufacturing certain short thioated DNA oligomers is estimated to be $50/g on the metric ton scale. This would allow large-scale preclinical pharmacological and toxicological studies and also, of course, clinical studies to be engaged. Futhermore, the following criteria should be met.

1   The drug should be stable after administration.
2   There should be a high probability of the drug entering target cells.
3   The drug should be retained in the *relevant* cell and not in irrelevant cells.
4   The metabolism of the drug *in vivo* should be reduced.
5   There should be a highly specific and efficient interaction with its target, e.g. mRNA.
6   An understanding of any non-sequence specific interaction with other molecules is required.
7   An investigation of safety and side-effects of the drug and any of its metabolic breakdown products should be conducted.
8   Its efficiency should be assessed *in vivo* and in the clinical setting.
9   The regulations involved in the development of any new drug should be adhered to.

Concerns such as these demand a rigorous understanding of the development of any drugs. I shall now describe the successes with these potential new drugs from laboratory cell culture experiments to the *in vivo* animal model systems that have taken place and have allowed the clinical trials to be authorised.

Earlier studies

As malignancy arises from a multistep process of oncogene activation or suppressor gene inactivation, it seems attractive to use antisense technology against genes such as *myc*, *ras* or *p53* (Heikkila *et al.*, 1987). Successful inhibition of the growth of leukaemia, breast and smooth muscle cells has been reported using DNA or RNA oligonucleotides, with claims of the induction of differentiation (Wickstrom *et al.*, 1988). These effects have often been shown to be dose dependent, and in some cases correlated with a reduction in oncogene mRNA and protein levels. Controls with sense, scrambled or mismatched sequences corroborated these results. There have been recorded and unrecorded failures in various laboratories, but often these involved different chemistries and variations in the oligomers used or lengths of the oligomer molecules or sequences targeted. With phosphothioated oligomers, side-effects were recorded, particularly at high concentrations of the oligomer.

The results recorded in other cell systems have been equally convincing, for example involving effects on protein kinase C or transforming growth factor-β1 (TGF-β1) mRNA molecules (Ahmad *et al.*, 1994; Dean *et al.*, 1994; Jun *et al.*, 1995). Indeed, techniques involving antisense have become the standard method of determining the function of any new oncogene or developmental process affected by a gene. Knockout strategies are a major advance in our understanding of gene function.

At the same time, the mechanisms of action of the antisense molecules were unravelled.

Mechanisms of action of antisense molecules

Once a DNA oligomer is bound to the RNA, forming a DNA–RNA hybrid, protein synthesis can be prevented by blocking either ribosomal binding or ribosomal progression. The hybrid may also provide a substrate for RNase H (Chiang *et al.*, 1991; Dean *et al.*, 1994), destabilise the 3′-untranslated end of the message with its poly(A) tail or disrupt mRNA splicing.

Oligonucleotides may also operate through triplex formation or by binding directly to specific proteins, the so-called aptameric reaction. The effects of aptamers are mediated by the complexing of a unique oligonucleotide and a unique protein and are dependent on oligomer sequence and backbone structure. Mixed oligonucleotides – chimaeras (see below) – may function via two of these mechanisms (Bergan, 1997).

Animal models and oligonucleotides

Following successful results with cell cultures, it was important to determine if down-regulation of genes in animal models could have biological effects. The aim of compartmentalised delivery in a clinical setting has seen application of these potential drugs to the skin, intravesical delivery to the bladder and intracranial injection for treatment of brain cancer. They have also been used in *ex vivo* bone marrow purges. The last approach allows small amounts of oligomer to be delivered systematically, eliminating side-effects.

At the same time, cellular uptake of oligomers, a notoriously poor process, can be improved in cell culture experiments by the use of liposomes or the addition of other groups to the oligomer. Uptake involves an association with the cell membrane and several proteins seem to be involved in this process (Beltinger *et al.*, 1995; Hawley and Gibson, 1996; Benimetskaya *et al.*, 1997). Different cell lines may have different receptor/oligomer relationships, but it seems to be agreed that adsorptive endocytosis is the key reaction in cellular uptake. Delivery by receptor-mediated endocytosis utilising oligomers conjugated to poly-lysine or complex glycopeptides with subsequent localisation in the liver or kidney of mice is under extensive study (Shreier *et al.*, 1994; Hangeland *et al.*, 1995; Thierry and Takle, 1995; Walker *et al.*, 1995). The localisation of oligomers in lysosomes, where enzyme digestion can take place, makes the targeting of the substrate in the nucleus or cytoplasm an inefficient process. Some research workers have resorted to microinjection or electroporation to introduce the antisense molecule. One group has been successful in targeting of the c-*myc* gene via an antisense mechanism or a protein tyrosine kinase by an aptameric mechanism following electroporation, achieving dramatic reductions in protein within 90 minutes. Specific effects on primary cultures of bone marrow left normal tissue functional but eliminated lymphoma cells following electroporation with c-*myc* antisense (Bergan, 1997).

In animal studies, targeting with DNA modified with methylphosphonate groups to a specific gene – c-*myc* – has been found to reduce lymphoma growth (Wickstrom, 1997). In this case, the antisense was injected through the tail vein. Continuous application to mice with a micro-osmotic pump also reduced the likelihood of developing tumours. Restenosis in pigs has also been inhibited with anti c-*myc* phosphorothioated antisense (Shi *et al.*, 1994). Wound healing and, in particular, the effects of scarring are influenced by the application to mice of antisense molecules against the growth factor TGF-β1. Similarly, c-H-*ras*-transformed cells, when treated with antisense and injected into mice, led to a great reduction in tumorigenesis (Gray *et al.*, 1993). *In vivo* tumour growth in mice has also been suppressed using antisense against the R1α gene, which encodes one of the regulatory units of protein kinase type A (Yoon *et al.*, 1997). Targeting the basic fibroblast growth factor and its receptor by antisense blocks the growth of melanoma cells

Table 7.1 Clinical trials in progress

Antisense DNA or ribozymes	Biological target
Ribozymes	HIV
Ribozymes	Brain tumours
Antisense	HIV
Antisense	Cytomegalovirus retinitis
Antisense	Human papilloma
Antisense	Crohn's disease
Antisense	Inflammatory/autoimmune disease
Antisense/ribozymes	Psoriasis
Antisense/ribozymes	Ulcerative colitis
Antisense/ribozymes	Rheumatoid arthritis
Antisense/ribozymes	Prevention of renal transplant rejection
Antisense/ribozymes	Non-Hodgkin's lymphoma
Antisense	Glioblastomas
Ribozymes	Hepatitis C and B

in mice (Wang and Becker, 1997). A cdk2 kinase oligomer prevents coronary arteriosclerosis in a mouse model (Suzuki *et al.*, 1997).

Antisense has also been used to prevent viral replication *in vitro* and in animal models. Successful results have been claimed with HIV and hepatitis B and C (Yu *et al.*, 1993; Temsamani and Agrawal, 1996).

In many of these cases, the actual mechanism leading to the biological effect was unclear.

Clinical trials

As a result of these successes, various clinical trials have been set up and are shown in Table 7.1.

Towards the next generation of antisense drugs

Initial experiments with antisense used phosphodiester oligomers. These were, however, unstable and subject to endonuclease and exonuclease digestion. Modifications of the backbone linkage were carried out, and this is still an active research arena (Figure 7.2).

Phosphorothioates are resistant to nucleases and easy to synthesise. They are, however, associated with non-specific side-effects (Krieg and Stein, 1995). Mixed backbone antisense molecules – so-called chimaeras – combining thioate and phosphodiester linkages (S and O) or

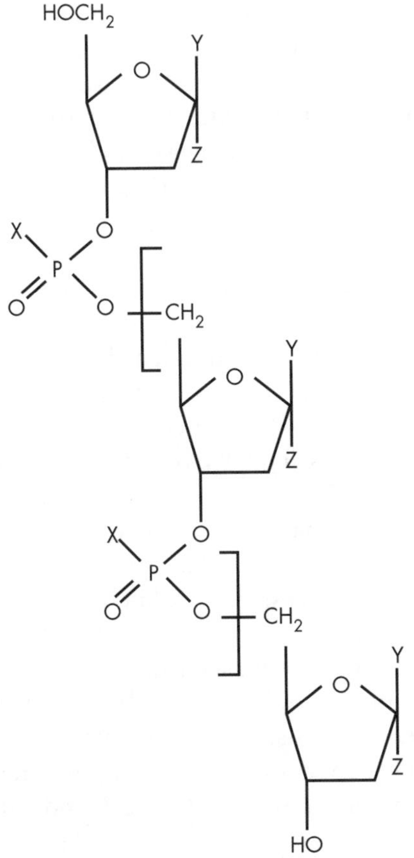

	X	Y	Z
Phosphodiester	O	A, G, C or T	H
Methylphosphonate	CH_2	A, G, C or T	H

Figure 7.2 Some modifications of oligodeoxynucleotides.

methylphosphonate (Me) and S or O linkages in the same molecule have been synthesised. These exhibit good stability, good hybridisation properties with the target mRNA, better entry into cells and less non-specific binding. Many other compounds have been produced, e.g. the peptide nucleic acid (PNA) backbone (Egholm *et al.*, 1992). This, for example, does not activate RNase H, but duplex and triplex PNA may bind to its target and block ribosome movement. Two current antisense favourites are the morpholino compounds (Summerton and Weller, 1993) and the phosphoroamidates (Froehler *et al.*, 1988).

One feature of all these compounds, both first- and second-generation compounds, is that toxicity and pharmacokinetic studies will be required to complement the delivery mechanisms which ensure they target the appropriate cells and reach the cytostol/nuclear components.

In vivo behaviour of oligonucleotides

Several of the oligonucleotides mentioned above have been administered to mice, rats, monkeys and humans. Thioated oligomers, for example, are well absorbed, rapidly distributed, show prolonged resistance to enzymatic attack in tissues and have broad peripheral tissue distribution (Agrawal *et al.*, 1995). They are cleared by metabolic processes over a prolonged period, more than 50% over 10 days, although others have claimed shorter half-lives (Zhang *et al.*, 1995; Temsamani *et al.*, 1997). The pattern is consistent across species, but humans probably metabolise them more slowly than rats. There are minimal differences between different sequences. Most studies acknowledge a preferential localisation of the oligonucleotides in the kidney and liver with a suggestion of *cell-specific* uptake, perhaps via scavenger receptor molecules. Where there have been differences they are explained by different routes of application, the chemical nature of the oligonucleotide, dose levels, species, age and size of animals, sample sizes, etc. Other criticisms include the analytical methods used to detect the oligomer and the programme used for pharmacokinetic analyses. The excretion of the antisense molecule takes place via the urine (Zhang *et al.*, 1995) or expired air (Cossum *et al.*, 1994) and this, it is claimed, depends on the method of labelling the compound. Comprehensive studies of the pharmacokinetics of various adapted oligomers are now in progress, and much of the research is not published. There is some general agreement, however.

The more stable the oligomer, the more it is taken up and the less it is eliminated (Agrawal *et al.*, 1997). Large sequences are retained particularly if they are end protected against enzymatic digestion (Crooke *et al.*, 1996). The oligomers and, in particular, the current favourite – the thioates – bind to plasma proteins and, therefore, are less available for cellular activity. It is also acknowledged that side-effects, e.g. elevation of liver enzyme levels in mice, can occur following the application of oligomers. Despite this, clinical trials with phosphorothioates in

HIV-infected individuals and leukaemic patients showed intact oligomer after 24 hours – 50% was excreted in the urine, increasing to 70% after 90 hours. There were no recorded side-effects that could not be managed medically. There are now some 15 clinical trials in operation with both antisense DNA (Crooke *et al.*, 1994; Bishop *et al.*, 1996; Calabretta *et al.*, 1996) and ribozymes (see below). Toxic effects are occasionally seen in mice that make it easier to control the pharmacological properties of the oligomers in human trials.

And finally

No review of antisense technology can be complete without the mention of another class of nucleotide molecules with particular targeting properties based partly on base pairing properties but also catalytic function – the ribozymes. These are RNA molecules with enzymatic activity that have great potential as therapeutic reagents since they can cleave mRNA molecules or effect the repair of mutant RNAs (Gibson, 1997).

They have been successful in many cell cultures and have overcome drug resistance and cell transformation by targeting the *mdr*-1 and Ha-*ras* mutant genes respectively (Koizumi *et al.*, 1992; Daly *et al.*, 1996). They are also effective against viral infections, e.g. HIV infection and hepatitis B and C in culture (Bauer *et al.*, 1997). They have also produced successful results in nude mice, in which they have been found to decrease drug resistance and reduce pleiotrophin levels in melanomas, and in humans, reducing metastatic spread of melanoma (Czubayko *et al.*, 1996) and restenosis following coronary artery angioplasty by acting on c-*myb* transcripts (Jarvis *et al.*, 1996). In the latter case it is recorded they are more successful than phosphorothioates. They also are effective on TNF-α, fibrillin and certain metalloproteinases, all of which suggests that they may be effective in clinical trials with patients with various conditions, e.g. Marfan syndrome (Kilpatrick *et al.*, 1996) or arthritis (Turck *et al.*, 1996). In theory, if a genetic cause is known to be associated with a disease, be it a mutation or a translocation, as in childhood myeloid leukaemia for example, ribozymes may be more effective than antisense DNA in eliminating the protein product. Many clinical trials with ribozymes are now under way; one surprising result is the finding that a specifically modified ribozyme can eliminate amelogenins, tissue-specific proteins that play a role in mammalian enamel biomineralisation, which is important in tooth formation.

Current trials into the effect of ribozymes on HIV using blood T lymphocytes or peripheral haemopoietic progenitor cells expressing CD34+ antigen have so far found no toxicity. Delivering ribozymes to cells by viral vector is likely to result in rapid advances. However, the problems already outlined associated with the use of antisense DNA molecules also apply to ribozymes, i.e. stability of uptake, pharmacokinetics. In many cases in which positive results have been achieved with ribozymes, the mechanism of action remains to be shown, particularly in animal experiments.

Conclusion

The field of antisense technology has recently become most popular as venture capital companies, mainly based in the USA, carry out the expensive synthesis and testing of oligomers of either DNA or RNA. Each company concentrates its research on one particular disease, be it Crohn's disease or psoriasis or particular cancers or viral infections. Experiments can be carried out quickly, many sites can be targeted, for example in the mRNA, many different methods can be used to introduce the molecules into the cell or organism and modifications to the oligonucleotide necessary to confer higher stability and improve uptake can be explored. A new DNA ribozyme that can also cleave RNA has been shown to have greater flexibility in selection of cleavage sites and, therefore, is able to target a wider range of mRNA sites (Kuwabara *et al.*, 1997). Antisense DNA modifications, particularly the N3′-P5′ phosphoroamidates (Gryaznov *et al.*, 1996), morpholine compounds (Summerton and Weller, 1993), the C_5 propyne pyrimidines (Wagner *et al.*, 1993) and 'clamping' adaptations to allow double-stranded DNA to form stable triplexes (Escudé *et al.*, 1996) are proving effective in cellular and preclinical studies.

The next few years should, with all the current activity, result in new breakthroughs and increase our armamentarium of drugs, but this time based on a rational design stemming from a knowledge of molecular biology. This should bring the advantages of more specific targeting and fewer side-effects.

References

Agrawal S, Temsamani J, Galbraith W, *et al.* (1995) Pharmacokinetics of antisense oligonucleotides. *Clin Pharmacokinet* 28: 7–16.

Agrawal S, Jiang Z, Zhao Q, et al. (1997) Mixed-backbone oligonucleotides as second generation antisense oligonucleotides: In vitro and in vivo studies. Proc Natl Acad Sci USA 94: 2620–2625.

Ahmad S, Mineta T, Martuza R L, et al. (1994) Antisense expression of protein kinase Cα inhibits the growth and tumorigenicity of human glioblastoma cells. Neurosurgery 35: 904–909.

Bauer G, Valdez P, Kearns K, et al. (1997) Inhibition of human immunodeficiency virus-1 (HIV-1) replication after transduction of granulocyte colony-stimulating factor-mobilised CD34(+) cells from HIV-1-infected donors using retroviral vectors containing anti-HIV-1 genes. Blood 89: 2259–2267.

Beltinger C, Saragovi H U, Smith R M, et al. (1995) Binding, uptake and intracellular trafficking of phosphorothioate-modified oligodeoxynucleotides. J Clin Invest 96: 1814–1823.

Benimetskaya L, Loike J, Khaled Z, et al. (1997) Mac-1 (CD11b/CD18) is a cell surface oligodeoxynucleotide binding protein. Nature Med 3: 414–420.

Bergan R C (1997) Ex vivo bone marrow purging with oligonucleotides. Antisense Nucleic Acid Drug Dev 7: 251–255.

Bishop M R, Iversen P L, Bayever E, et al. (1996) Phase I trial of an antisense oligonucleotide OL(1) p53 in hematologic malignancies. J Clin Oncol 14: 1320–1326.

Calabretta B, Skorski T, Ratajczak M Z, et al. (1996) Antisense strategies in the treatment of leukemias. Semin Oncol 23: 78–87.

Chiang M-Y, Chan H, Zounes M A, et al. (1991) Antisense oligonucleotides inhibit intercellular adhesion molecule 1 expression by two distinct mechanisms. J Biol Chem 266: 18162–18171.

Cossum P A, Truong L, Oens S R, et al. (1994) Pharmacokinetics of a ^{14}C-labeled phosphorothioate oligonucleotide, ISIS 2105, after intradermal administration to rats. J Pharmacol Exp Ther 269: 89–94.

Crooke S T, Grillone L R, Tendolkar A, et al. (1994) A pharmacokinetic evaluation of ^{14}C-labeled afovirsen sodium in patients with genital warts. Clin Pharmacol Ther 56: 641–646.

Crooke S T, Graham M J, Zuckerman J E, et al. (1996) Pharmacokinetic properties of several novel oligonucleotide analogs in mice. J Pharmacol Exp Ther 277: 923–937.

Czubayko F, Schulte A M, Berchem G J, et al. (1996) Melanoma angiogenesis and metastasis modulated by ribozyme targeting of the secreted growth-factor pleiotrophin. Proc Natl Acad Sci USA 93: 14753–14758.

Daly C, Coyle S, McBride S, et al. (1996) mdr1 ribozyme mediated reversal of the multi-drug resistant phenotype in human lung cell lines. Cytotechnology 19: 199–205.

Dean N M, McKay R, Condon T P, et al. (1994) Inhibition of protein kinase C-α expression in human A549 cells by antisense oligonucleotides inhibits induction of intercellular adhesion molecule 1 (1CAM-1) mRNA by phorbol esters. J Biol Chem 269: 16416–16424.

Egholm M, Buchardt O, Nielsen P, et al. (1992) Peptide nucleic acids (PNA). Oligonucleotide analogues with an achiral peptide backbone. J Am Chem Soc 114: 1895–1897.

Escudé C, Giovannangeli C, Sun J-S, et al. (1996) Stable triple helices formed by oligonucleotide N3′→P5′-phosphoramidates inhibit transcription elongation. *Proc Natl Acad Sci USA* 93: 4365–4369.

Froehler B, Ng P, Matteucci M (1988) Phosphoramidate analogues of DNA: synthesis and thermal stability of heteroduplexes. *Nucleic Acids Res* 16: 4831–4839.

Gibson I, ed. (1997) *Antisense and Ribozyme Methodology.* London: Chapman & Hall, 1–79.

Gray G, Hebel D, Hernandez O, *et al.* (1993) Antisense DNA inhibition of c-H*aras* induced tumor growth in nude mice. *Cancer Res* 53: 577–580.

Gryaznov S, Skorski T, Cucco C, *et al.* (1996) Oligonucleotide N3′-P5′ phosphoroamidates as antisense agent. *Nucleic Acids Res* 24: 1508–1514.

Hangeland J J, Levis J T, Lee Y C, *et al.* (1995) Cell-type specific and ligand-specific enhancement of cellular uptake of oligodeoxynucleoside methylphosphonates covalently linked with a neoglycopeptide, YEE (ah-Ga1NAc)$_3$. *Bioconj Chem* 6: 695–701.

Hawley P, Gibson I (1996) Interaction of oligodeoxynucleotides with mammalian cells. *Antisense Nucleic Acid Drug Dev* 6: 197–206.

Heikkila R, Schwab G, Wickstrom E, *et al.* (1987) A *c-myc* antisense oligodeoxynucleotide inhibits entry into S phase but not progress from G_0 to G_1. *Nature* 328: 445–449.

Jarvis T C, Alby L J, Beaudry A A, *et al.* (1996) Inhibition of vascular smooth muscle cell-proliferation by ribozymes that cleave *c-myc* messenger-RNA. *RNA* 2: 419–428.

Jun C D, Choi B M, Kim S U, *et al.* (1995) Downregulation of transforming growth factor-β gene expression by antisense oligodeoxynucleotides increases recombinant interferon-g-induced nitric oxide synthesis in murine peritoneal macrophages. *Immunology* 85: 114–119.

Kilpatrick M W, Phylactou L A, Godfrey M, *et al.* (1996) Delivery of a hammerhead ribozyme specifically down-regulated the production of fibrillin-1 by cultured dermal fibroblasts. *Hum Mol Genet* 5: 1939–1944.

Koizumi M, Kamiya H, Ohtsuka E (1992) Ribozymes designed to inhibit transformation of NIH3T3 cells by the activated c-Ha-*ras* gene. *Gene* 117: 179–184.

Krieg A, Stein C (1995) Phosphorothioate oligodeoxynucleotides: Antisense or antiprotein? *Antisense Res Dev* 5: 241.

Kuwabara T, Warashima M, Tanabet T, *et al.* (1997) Comparison of the specificities and catalytic activities of hammerhead ribozymes and DNA enzyme with respect to the cleavage of Bcr-Abl chimeric L6 (b2a2) mRNA. *Nucleic Acids Res* 25: 3074–3081.

Schreier H, Moran P, Caras I W (1994) Targeting of liposomes to cells expressing CD4 using glycosylphosphatidylinositol-anchored gp120. *J Biol Chem* 269: 9090–9098.

Shi Y, Fard A, Galeo A, *et al.* (1994) Transcatheter delivery of *c-myc* antisense oligomers reduces neointimal formation in a porcine model of coronary artery balloon injury. *Circulation* 90: 944–951.

Stephenson M L, Zamecnik P C (1978) Inhibition of Rous sarcoma viral RNA translation by a specific oligodeoxynucleotide. *Proc Natl Acad Sci USA* 75: 285–288.

Stull R A, Szoka F C Jr (1995) Antigene, ribozyme and aptamer nucleic acid drugs: progress and prospects. *Pharmacol Res* 12: 465–483.

Summerton J, Weller D (1993) Uncharged morpholino-based polymers having phosphorus-containing chiral intersubunit linkages. *US Patent 5*: 185, 444.

Suzuki J-I, Isobe M, Morishita R, *et al.* (1997) Prevention of graft coronary arteriosclerosis by antisense cdk2 kinase oligonucleotide. *Nature Med* 8: 900–903.

Temsamani J, Agrawal S (1996) Antisense oligonucleotide as antiviral agents. In: de Clerq E, ed. *Advances in Antiviral Drug Design*, Vol. 2. Greenwich, CT: JAI Press, 1–39.

Temsamani J, Roskey A, Chaix C, *et al.* (1997) *In vivo* metabolic profile of a phosphorothioate oligodeoxynucleotide. *Antisense Nucl Acid Drug Dev* 7: 159–165.

Thierry A R, Takle GB (1995) Liposomes as a delivery system for antisense and ribozyme compounds. In: Akhtar S, ed. *Delivery Strategies for Antisense Oligonucleotide Therapeutics*. Boca Raton, FL: CRC Press, 199–221.

Turck J, Pollack A S, Lee L K, *et al.* (1996) Matrix metalloproteinase 2 (gelatinase A) regulates glomerular mesengial cell proliferation and differentiation *J Biol Chem* 271: 15074–15083.

Wagner R, Matteucci M, Lewis J, *et al.* (1993) Antisense gene inhibition by oligonucleotides containing C-5 propyne pyrimidines. *Science* 260: 1510–1513.

Walker I, Irwin W J, Akhtar S (1995) Improved cellular delivery of antisense oligonucleotides using transferrin receptor antibody–oligonucleotide conjugates. *Pharm Res* 12: 1548–1553.

Wang Y, Becker D (1997) Antisense targeting of basic fibroblast growth factor and fibroblast growth factor receptor in human melanoma blocks intratumour angiogenesis and tumour growth. *Nature Med* 8: 887–893.

Wickstrom E L, ed. (1991) *Prospects for Antisense Nucleic Acid Therapy of Cancer and AIDS*. New York: Wiley-Liss.

Wickstrom E L (1997) Antisense *c-myc* Inhibition of lymphoma growth. *Antisense Nucl Acid Drug Dev* 7: 225–228.

Wickstrom E L, Bacon T A, Gonzalez A, *et al.* (1988) Human promyelocytic leukemia HL-60 cell proliferation and *c-myc* protein expression are inhibited by an antisense pentadecadeoxynucleotide targeted against *c-myc* mRNA. *Proc Natl Acad Sci USA* 85: 1028–1032.

Yoon S Cho-Chung, Nesterova M, Kondrashin A, *et al.* (1997) Antisense-protein kinase A: A single-gene-based therapeutic approach. *Antisense Nucl Acid Drug Dev* 7: 217–223.

Yu M, Ojwang J, Yamada O, *et al.* (1993) A hairpin ribozyme inhibits expression of diverse strains of human immunodeficiency virus type 1. *Proc Natl Acad Sci USA* 90: 6340–6344.

Zamecnik P C, Stephenson M L (1978) Inhibition of Rous sarcoma virus replication and transformation by a specific oligodeoxynucleotide. *Proc Natl Acad Sci USA* 75: 280–284.

Zhang X, Lu Z, Diasio R B, *et al.* (1995) Plasma- and serum-protein binding of antisense oligodeoxynucleotide phosphorothioates in experimental animals and humans. *Proc Am Assoc Cancer Res* 36: 411.

8

Potential use of transgenic animals in health and disease

Gavin Brooks

Transgenic manipulation is the process whereby genes from one species are introduced into the germ line of another distantly related species for the purpose of either producing large and relatively cheap amounts of the gene product or to study the physiological consequences of altering the gene. Although there are some similarities between transgenic technology and gene therapy (Chapter 6), the major difference between the two technologies is that in gene therapy the therapeutic gene is transferred to the somatic cells only (i.e. all cells in the body except the germ cells or their precursors), whereas transgenic organisms express the foreign gene both in somatic cells and in germline cells. Thus, in transgenic organisms, the genetic changes are conserved in any offspring according to the general rules of Mendelian inheritance. The use of animal organs, whether they are obtained from genetically engineered (transgenic) or normal animals, for transplantation into humans (xenotransplantation) has become the subject of much debate in recent months. One of the major issues, apart from ethical ones, appears to be the possibility that viruses from the donor organ can infect cells in the recipient human host. Despite these issues, the possibility of developing transgenic animals for medical research remains a valuable approach to understanding the mechanisms of disease. Theoretically, transgenic technology enables the introduction of virtually any gene into any organism, and the technique has considerable potential in a number of areas, including farming, agriculture, pharmaceuticals (including the production of drugs and the generation of models of human disease) and surgery. This chapter describes the basic methodology and current pharmaceutical and non-pharmaceutical uses of transgenic organisms and discusses their relevance to medicine. Finally, as mentioned above, a number of ethical and other considerations have to be considered before transgenesis can be used routinely and these will be discussed also.

Approaches used for the production of transgenic animals

Until a few years ago, it was not possible to study certain disease processes adequately because of the lack of suitable and relevant mammalian model systems. However, recent and rapid advances in mouse genetics have enabled this animal system to be manipulated such that various human disease phenotypes can be mimicked in the mouse by applying transgenic technology. Until the advent of such mouse systems, bacteria were used routinely as vehicles for producing large quantities of foreign genes because they multiply rapidly, thereby ensuring that large quantities of the required gene product can be obtained in a relatively short period of time. However, bacteria do not represent good models of human disease and so more suitable mammalian systems were sought. The mouse has been the mammalian species of choice for developing transgenic technology (although more recently the technique has been applied to a variety of species, including rats, rabbits, sheep and goats) for a number of reasons, including (a) the genetic make-up of the mouse is well characterised and is the best understood of all mammals; (b) the mouse and human genomes contain approximately the same number of genes, have the same size genomes and display their genes in the same order on their chromosomes; (c) the mouse has been used in genetic research since Mendelian times; and (d) mice are small, have a short gestation period with a large number of offspring and breed easily.

The ability to introduce, in a stable manner, foreign DNA into the germ line of a mammalian species was not developed until the late 1970s (Jaenisch, 1977). Mice were the first species to be engineered to carry a foreign gene, and these animals were derived by microinjecting simian virus 40 (SV40) DNA into mouse blastocysts (Jaenisch and Mintz, 1974). However, these genetically manipulated animals failed to demonstrate integration of the inserted SV40 gene into their germ cells and expression of the gene was restricted to somatic cells. However, in 1977 the first successful germline transmission of foreign DNA was achieved when mouse embryos were exposed to infectious Moloney leukaemia retrovirus (Jaenisch, 1977). Since that time, numerous reports have appeared in the literature demonstrating stable expression of a variety of genes in transgenic mouse lines.

Methods for the introduction of foreign genes into animals

Three methods are used currently to introduce foreign genes into recipient animals. These are described below.

Direct microinjection of DNA into the pronucleus of fertilised eggs

This is the most successful and widely used method for producing transgenic mice. Initially, the DNA of interest is microinjected into either the female or male pronucleus. This leads to a random integration of the DNA into the genome of the injected egg such that it will subsequently be distributed between both somatic and germline cells. Following microinjection of the DNA, up to 35 injected embryos are reimplanted into the oviducts of pseudopregnant foster mothers and allowed to develop to term (Figure 8.1). The pseudopregnant foster mothers are produced by mating females in natural oestrus with vasectomised or genetically sterile male animals. As a consequence, the reproductive tract of these mated females will then become receptive for transferred embryos, even though their own unfertilised eggs will degenerate (Hogan *et al.*, 1986). The number of embryos injected into the oviducts of the foster mother is so high because the rate of implantation is low, with only 8–10 littermates being produced on average. As the microinjected DNA is distributed between both somatic and germline cells, not only will the developing embryo itself express the inserted gene in all cells of its body, but any progeny from the mature organism also will express the gene. At birth the pups are screened [e.g. by Southern analysis (see Chapter 1) of tail biopsies] to identify those animals with gametes originating from the inserted DNA (i.e. germline transgenics). Those animals that have developed from injected eggs are termed 'founder' animals. As soon as it has been determined that a founder animal is transgenic, it usually is mated to begin establishing a transgenic line. In theory, most transgenic founders should transmit the foreign gene to 50% of their offspring, although in reality up to 20% of transgenic founders transmit the transgene at a lower frequency (e.g. 5–10% instead of 50%) (Hogan *et al.*, 1986). Furthermore, problems occur if the transgenic male is sterile or semisterile, which is not an uncommon occurrence. It is essential that offspring from the second generation of transgenic animals (and all subsequent generations) are screened by tail biopsies for the presence of the transgene as it is possible that the transgene will segregate into only one of the germ cells of the founder animal, which would result in the transgene not being passed onto all offspring. Despite these limitations, direct microinjection has the advantage of being able to generate transgenic lines that express most genes in a predictable manner, and it has been reported that >25% of pups derived from microinjected embryos will express the transgene (Field, 1991). However, one disadvantage of this method is that it has to be carried out specifically at the pronucleus stage since it cannot be used to

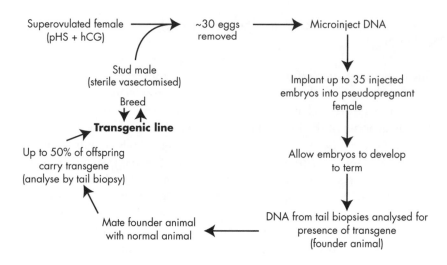

Figure 8.1 Establishment of a transgenic line. hCG, human chorionic gonadotrophin; pHS, pregnant mare's serum.

introduce genes into cells at later stages of development, i.e. after the zygote has divided.

Retroviral infection

This technique has been described in detail in Chapter 6 and so the methodology involved will not be discussed further here. One advantage of this method for producing transgenic animals is that it enables genes to be transferred into preimplantation stage embryos (e.g. during the first 5 days of development in the mouse) by exposing them to concentrated stocks of infecting virus or co-cultivating them on monolayers of virus-producing cells. More recently, methods have been devised to introduce infecting virus into post-implantation embryos between days 8 and 12 of gestation (Hogan *et al.*, 1986). Although this technique enables the infection of cells from many somatic tissues, germ cells are infected with low frequency. However, this approach is one of the only methods available currently to generate certain transgenic species since the pronuclei of certain species, e.g. chicken, cannot be microinjected with foreign DNA.

The main advantage of using retroviral infection is the technical ease with which genes can be introduced into the embryos at various stages of development. However, one major problem with the approach is the size limitation of the introduced DNA (up to 7 kb of DNA can be inserted), which is not sufficient for some large genes. This problem, coupled with the fact that levels of expression of the transgene in germline cells by this method is low, means that retroviral infection is not used routinely in the production of transgenic animals.

Embryonic stem (ES) cells

ES cells serve as the starting point for all cell lineages in the body since they are multipotent, i.e. they are capable of differentiating into a variety of different cell types depending upon the availability of certain growth factors and/or cytokines. ES cells are being used increasingly in the production of transgenic animals because they can be established in a tissue culture dish from normal 3.5-day post-coital explanted blastocysts (i.e. the eight- to 16-cell cluster of cells forming the early embryo). Once established in culture, DNA is introduced into ES cells by a variety of transfection methods, e.g. electroporation, calcium phosphate precipitation, lipofection or direct microinjection (Brooks, 1994, and Chapter 6). Those ES cells carrying the transgene are selected in tissue culture and injected into normal explanted host blastocysts, where they can colonise the embryo and contribute to the germ line of the resultant transgenic animal. These 'ES cell blastocysts' are reimplanted into the uterus of a pseudopregnant foster mother, where they develop and behave as a normal blastocyst, and the embryos are allowed to develop to term. The major advantage of this approach is that large numbers of transgenic animals can be generated once an ES cell has been transfected stably. The only real drawback to this method is the technical difficulty associated with manipulating the embryo and the subsequent maintenance of the cells in culture. In addition, difficulties also may be associated with optimising the efficiency of transfection, which can vary depending upon the gene of interest.

Choice of animal species for transgenic technology

Theoretically, virtually any gene can be introduced into the germ line of any organism, although certain practical considerations restrict the total number of genes/species that can be manipulated. For instance, the chosen species should ideally breed rapidly and produce a large number of offspring. In addition, it should be easy to keep free from viral infections. Husbandry costs and time to reach maturity also should be considered when selecting a suitable animal model. As mentioned above, the mouse is the best mammalian system for studying genetic contributions to human disease since they are genetically the best characterised mammalian system; they are easy to breed; they have a short generation time; and there is a wide availability of inbred strains (Breslow, 1993). However, the mouse is not necessarily ideal for studying all human disorders, and one argument against using this species is the small size of the animal. Rats have certain advantages over mice in that they are of a larger size, thus making surgical and physiological manipulations easier, and there are now a number of literature reports describing the production of transgenic rats (e.g. Field, 1991; Crabbe *et al.*, 1994). Baboons are even better suited as a model system to compare with the human situation, especially if the animal's organs are to be used for transplantation (see below). However, baboons are slow breeders and are difficult to keep free from viral infections. Pigs, by contrast, are about the same size as humans, have a similar physiology and can be bred more easily than baboons in sterile conditions and are possibly the most promising source of transgenic organs suitable for transplantation into humans (see below). A further consideration is whether the transferred gene will be active in the transgenic species. For example, human renin will not process mouse or rat angiotensinogen (Field, 1991). Thus, if one wishes to increase angiotensin II levels in a transgenic mouse, there is no point in overexpressing human renin.

Finally, there is considerable commercial interest in developing certain other transgenic species, e.g. cows, sheep, goats and horses, in order to obtain certain desirable characteristics, e.g. increased meat–fat ratio in beef cattle and muscle or for improving speed in racehorses.

Gene knockouts (gene targeting)

The majority of early transgenic lines were produced by overexpressing a normal gene that, before insertion into the animal, was either non-functional or only partially functional. This is commonly referred to as a gain-of-function approach. An alternative approach, developed more recently, is to prevent the expression of a gene by knocking it out. 'Knockouts' are produced by transfecting ES cells with a mutated copy of the gene of interest. This replaces the endogenous gene by the process of homologous recombination. This is an extremely powerful technique for studying the effects of individual genes and complex developmental processes and has proven useful for investigating certain human diseases since knockout mice display symptoms that are very similar to those observed in people who lack the same gene. Indeed, a biotechnology company called Lexicon Genetics in Texas, USA, is currently creating a bank of more than 500 000 mutant mice, each of which will contain a single defective gene (Coghlan, 1996). The aim of the company is to make available strains of mice that are defective in one of all the 100 000 genes found in the human genome, thereby enabling geneticists to study the function of 'silenced' genes.

One of the major problems with the knockout approach has been tissue and/or cell specific inactivation of the gene of interest. In many of these studies, the embryo fails to develop or the pup dies soon after birth because the knocked out gene is essential for development. Recently, Klaus Rajewsky, an immunologist at the University of Cologne, has achieved cell-specific inactivation of the gene for DNA polymerase β in the T cells of mice (Barinaga, 1994). Although this is the first report of such specificity in transgenic animals, the method should be generally applicable to other cell types and genes.

Use of transgenic animals in medicine

Research

The methods now available for introducing foreign DNA into fertilised eggs have led to the development of a number of transgenic animal models for human diseases, including cancer, AIDS, diabetes, atherosclerosis and psoriasis. A number of possibilities now exist for studying gene expression during development, and for following the consequences of altering or blocking specific gene products or for understanding and rectifying inherited defects and childhood cancers. Good animal models of human diseases such as CF were, until recently, very rare. Indeed, those chronic human diseases that cause degeneration of brain and the nervous system have been among the most difficult to study, mainly because there are few, if any, small animal models that accurately mimic the pathology and clinical features of the disease. However, in the past 2–3 years, transgenic mouse lines that mimic the symptoms seen in such human diseases have been generated. For example, a transgenic mouse model for CF was developed recently by introducing the *CFTR* gene into an ES cell system (Dorin *et al.*, 1992;

Ratcliff *et al.*, 1993), and such animal models of human disease can be used to study possible mechanisms that lead to the disease and provide a valid model system for the development and testing of therapies, e.g. for CF patients.

In another example, transgenic mice expressing the product of the gene for human apolipoprotein(a), elevated levels of which are associated with an increased risk for atherosclerosis and its manifestations, i.e. myocardial infarction, stroke and restenosis, have been produced. These transgenic animals are more susceptible than control mice to the development of lipid-staining lesions in the aorta (Lawn *et al.*, 1992) and will provide a good model with which to study the mechanisms associated with atherosclerosis. Other atherosclerotic models are available following the production of knockout mice lacking the genes for various lipoprotein transport proteins, including apolipoproteins, processing proteins, e.g. lipoprotein lipase, and receptors, e.g. low-density lipoprotein receptor (Breslow, 1993). These animals will provide good model systems with which to study various aspects of atherosclerosis.

An American biotechnology company has already produced and patented an oncomouse that has been genetically engineered to develop cancer within a few months of birth (Moore, 1993). While this model will enable scientists to study in more detail the early events that lead to cancer – in addition to providing a system for testing novel anti-cancer drugs – it has led to some concerns among animal welfare campaigners. These campaigners have expressed concern that animal suffering should be minimised in research and not increased, as in the case of the oncomouse.

Very recently, a transgenic mouse model for studying fatal amyotrophic lateral sclerosis or Lou Gehrig's disease was reported (Gurney *et al.*, 1994). This disease causes degeneration of motor neurones in the cortex, brainstem and spinal cord and produces complete paralysis followed by death. A transgenic model for this disease was produced by introducing a mutant gene for Cu/Zn superoxide dismutase into the germ line of mice. This model should help in elucidation of the underlying mechanisms involved in this disorder.

Organ transplantation (xenotransplantation)

One of the most controversial advances in surgery in recent years has been the potential use of genetically modified animal organs (especially derived from pigs) for transplantation into humans. Such is the expected need for animal organs that the Cambridge-based biotechnology company Imutran is in the process of producing genetically modified pigs in a programme of research that will hopefully lead to transplantable organs. While animal tissues and products have been used in surgical procedures for many years, e.g. pig aortic valves in valve replacement surgery, the proposed transplantation of intact organs is more recent, and a number of research teams and biotechnology companies are currently exploring the potential benefits of such an approach. The major thrust of this research is centred upon the development of transgenic pig hearts suitable for transplantation into humans. The heart is a priority for such research since it is not possible to keep the heart alive by dialysis as is the case for some other organs, e.g. liver and kidney. The pig heart is ideal for this procedure because it is similar in size and blood vessel composition to the human heart. Indeed, the availability of animal hearts would reduce the current waiting list for heart transplants considerably as, in Britain alone, at least 25% of heart patients requiring a transplant die while waiting for a suitable donor heart to become available (Concar, 1994).

The transplantation of animal organs into humans is not without problems, however. One of the major problems associated with transplanting an animal organ into a human recipient is the hyperacute rejection of the animal's organ in transplant patients. In an effort to minimise these risks, scientists in Cambridge, UK, have recently produced a transgenic pig line by microinjecting human DNA encoding the gene for decay accelerating factor (DAF) into a pig embryo (Concar, 1994). The protein product of this gene, i.e. DAF, prevents hyperacute rejection of the pig's organs in transplant patients. The hope is that the transgene for DAF will make the pig organs compatible with the human immune system. The future may provide the possibility of every individual having their own transgenic pig, purpose built to avoid tissue rejection, such that a ready supply of replacement organs would be available should the human counterparts fail due to disease or accident. The production of a personalised transgenic pig would be essential since use of organs from a generic pig would not be feasible owing to the immune responses that would be initiated when the organ was transplanted into the recipient human patient.

The gene knockout approach is currently being developed in pigs, which are being engineered to act as organ donors for human recipients (Concar, 1994). As mentioned above, one potential problem with using tissue from another organism is the hyperacute rejection of the transplanted organ. Antibodies produced by the recipient's immune system play a significant role in this rejection. Recently, it has been shown that a major target of these antibodies, especially against porcine transplanted organs, is gal(α-1,3)gal, a sugar found on the surfaces of pig epithelial cells (Concar, 1994). One approach to this problem has been to disable or 'knock out' the pig gene encoding one of the enzymes needed to tether gal(α-1,3)gal to the host cell surface. Although elimination of the hyperacute rejection response is essential if the patient is to survive, this therapy will not reduce any longer term rejection responses in the transplanted organ, e.g. from T cells. Furthermore, it may not be possible to suppress the body's natural immune response with immunosuppressant drugs sufficiently when animal organs are transplanted into human patients as immune responses may be more severe than when human–human transplantation is used. This very sophisticated technology is still very much in its infancy and, although the future potential of this approach is enormous, current progress is extremely slow because of numerous technical problems.

Other examples of animal tissues being used for transplantation into humans include the transplantation of dopaminergic neurones from the brains of pig fetuses into the brains of human patients suffering from Parkinson's disease (Brown, 1997; Isacson and Breakefield, 1997) and the transplantation of mouse cells that have been genetically modified to produce a retrovirus that expresses the thymidine kinase (*tk*) gene into the brains of humans suffering from glioma (Isacson and Breakefield, 1997). When these patients are treated with the drug ganciclovir, those cells that express the *tk* gene are killed selectively. As normal, non-malignant neurones do not divide, they do not take up the retrovirus and so are not killed by ganciclovir. Both examples described above currently are in phase I clinical trials in the USA. Other researchers are investigating the potential use of genetically modified fish as donors for pancreatic cells to be transplanted into children suffering from diabetes (Mackenzie, 1996). In this example, scientists in Canada have been investigating the possibility of using islets of Langerhans cells derived from the pancreas of the freshwater fish *Telapia* that have been genetically modified to secrete human insulin for transplantation into the livers of humans who have had to have their pancreas removed for various reasons. Although this is a rare procedure, it is performed when a patient is very ill, and currently islets of Langerhans cells from three donor humans are required per recipient. Thus, the advent of an animal source for these cells could result in many more lives being saved. Unfortunately, the pig is not a good candidate for the production of such genetically modified cells as 10 pigs would be required per human recipient and animals need to be reared in sterile conditions for 2 years, thereby making production costs prohibitive. The use of *Telapia* would provide large amounts of pancreatic cells relatively cheaply, and recent studies have shown that islet cells can be isolated easily from these fish and that they can be successfully transplanted into mice and rats and produce insulin in response to changing blood sugar levels. Scientists hope that in the near future fish expressing human insulin can be produced in sufficient numbers such that transplantation of fish islet cells into children suffering from diabetes will bring to an end the need for daily injections of insulin for millions of children suffering from this disease.

Although the potential for using animal organs for transplantation into humans is immense, one potentially serious problem has recently come to light. This relates to the possibility of endogenous retroviruses, which are harmless in the natural host, crossing species and causing disease in the new host. Indeed, it is known that viruses can cross species and cause disease in the new host, e.g. AIDS and bovine spongiform encephalitis, although usually such transmitted organisms are dealt with by the body's defences. Recently, researchers have shown that pigs carry a virus that can infect human cells (Brown, 1997), raising concerns about the use of pig organs for human transplantation. As a result of these findings, the American Food and Drug Administration (FDA) and the Centers for Disease Control (CDC) in Atlanta, USA, have published guidelines for the use of animal organs in human transplants. They recommend that animals are screened for disease, that samples of tissue are archived, that local review boards are set up to evaluate the risks of infectious disease and that individuals who receive organs are monitored afterwards; however, it is not clear which diseases should be monitored. Furthermore, in January 1997, the British government gave its support to continued research into transplantation of pig organs into humans. However, it stipulated that clinical trials using this technology should be banned until further research shows that such transplants are safe and that patients will benefit (Williams, 1997), and further research was deemed necessary into the potential for new human diseases arising from exposure to pig pathogens. The British government has established the UK Xenotransplantation Interim Regulatory Authority to control developments in the field of organ transplants between species while a full legal framework is developed. The Authority has agreed that the transplantation of pig organs is ethically acceptable but has ruled out the use of primates as a source of donor organs. It has stated that primates should be used only for xenotransplantation research and then only when there is no suitable alternative method of obtaining critical information. Obviously, when animal-to-human organ transplants are undertaken, careful monitoring of blood samples by PCR (Chapter 5) and serology will be essential to assess the possible generation of infectious retroviruses. Furthermore, it is crucial that recipients are not of child-bearing age and that they should not donate their blood or organs to others. Other precautionary measures that could be taken include immunising recipients against host retroviruses.

Pharmaceuticals

Transgenic animals are now being developed for use in the pharmaceutical industry to assist with drug development, e.g. anti-AIDS drugs. One problem with the *in vivo* testing of agents for the treatment of AIDS is that only two available animal species are sensitive to HIV infection: the gibbon and the chimpanzee. Gibbons are not permitted to be used in biomedical research and, although chimpanzees can be used, they are expensive and only can be used in limited numbers. However, a transgenic mouse system for the easy *in vitro* evaluation of new anti-human HIV type 1 drugs or therapies designed specifically to target a viral trans-activator protein called TAT or long terminal repeat (LTR) functions has recently been introduced (Mehtali *et al.*, 1992) (an LTR is a sequence of DNA that can control expression of a gene which is attached to it). The recent development of this transgenic mouse model will provide the large numbers of small animals required for the testing of potential anti-AIDS drugs.

Recently, a number of genetic animal models of alcohol and drug abuse have been developed (Crabbe *et al.*, 1994). The large majority of these are mouse models, including high/low ethanol withdrawal mice and alcohol-preferring versus non-preferring mice, although some rat models are available, e.g. alcohol ataxia non-tolerant and tolerant rats. Although not directly transgenic, these models will enable genes which are thought to play a role in alcohol and other drug abuse to be identified.

The human gene for α_1-antitrypsin, which is required to treat hereditary emphysema, has been inserted into the germ line of sheep (Concar, 1994). This enzyme is normally very expensive when produced in the laboratory but is significantly cheaper when extracted from the milk of the transgenic sheep. A further example of a transgenic sheep model secretes human factor IX in its milk. This serves as a valuable source of this otherwise expensive clotting agent for haemophiliacs. In a similar manner, a transgenic cow has been produced that secretes human α-lactalbumin into its milk (Anon, 1997). Alpha-lactalbumin is a protein that is found in significant amounts in human breast milk and serves as a rich and balanced source of amino acids that are required by newborn babies. The transgenic cow currently produces 2.4 g/l of milk compared with 2.7 g/l in human breast milk, although it is anticipated that, when mature, the cow will produce 10 000 litres of milk per year. Accordingly, the biotechnology company PPL Therapeutics in Blacksburg, Virginia, USA, is planning to market the protein in a purified form, which then could be added to powdered milks for premature babies. Although the potential benefit of generating genetically modified sheep and cows is enormous, the procedure is currently limited because it is laborious, time-consuming and expensive.

Other uses of transgenic technology

Crop production

There now exists the technology to modify lipid, starch and protein storage reserves in seeds, impart pest/virus resistance and/or create modified plants that tolerate extreme habitats, e.g. salt marshes or waterlogged soil. Furthermore, it is possible to alter the nutritive content of a plant or to increase its resistance to disease. Usually, genes are introduced into plants by using plant cells which have had their cell walls removed to produce protoplasts. Foreign DNA is then introduced into these protoplasts by conventional transfection or infection methods (see Brooks, 1994, for details). The transfected protoplasts are encouraged to reform their cell walls, divide and regenerate into a new transgenic plant (Alberts *et al.*, 1989). This technique has been used to produce transgenic *Sorghum* plants (Casas *et al.*, 1993). Sorghum (*Sorghum bicolor* L. Moench) is an important cereal crop typically grown in areas where soil moisture is unsuitable for maize. It is a primary staple diet for those who live in the semiarid regions of Africa and Asia. In the West, sorghum is commonly used as a feedstuff for livestock. Transgenic sorghum plants have been produced by introducing the gene encoding phosphinothricin acetyltransferase into protoplasts. The resultant plants are both drought resistant and herbicide resistant (Casas *et al.*, 1993). To date, transgenic systems have been developed for other cereal crops of major agricultural importance, including maize, oat, rice and wheat (Casas *et al.*, 1993, and references therein).

A further example of transgenic technology being used in agriculture has been reported recently in the USA, where a gene has been inserted into tomatoes to prevent the fruit from going soft and mushy as it ripens (Moore, 1993). Other transgenic approaches currently being developed include the overexpression of carotenoids in tomatoes and other edible plants since these antioxidants have been shown to reduce the incidence of certain diseases, e.g. cardiovascular disease (Bramley, 1997). Thus, individuals would have to eat less of these transgenic plants to obtain a significant concentration of carotenoids in their diet.

Farming

Transgenic technology is currently used in farming either to alter the growth rate in farm animals or to alter the body composition to change the fat–meat ratio (Moore, 1993). Obviously, the concept of producing better quality livestock is not a new one, so why are farmers bothering to produce such transgenic animals? The reasons are simply that conventional breeding programmes are very slow and the results unpredictable and often poor. Transgenic manipulation of a farm animal enables a single gene to be chosen and inserted into the organism, therefore greatly increasing the chances of a successful outcome.

The gene knockout approach has been used in fish, in which two genes have been independently introduced into carp (Moore, 1993). One of these genes encodes for growth hormone and another encodes the gene for an 'antifreeze' protein that will enable fish to survive in cold waters. Obvious problems exist with such genetic manipulations as deliberate or accidental release of such transgenic fish into the open environment could result in huge changes in the native populations of fish, with possible consequences for other animals and plants.

Ethical considerations

As illustrated above, the potential uses of transgenic organisms are extensive. However, as is the case with any form of genetic manipulation, it is essential that guidelines are drawn up and that all persons involved adhere to these absolutely. One particular problem with this type of work is that in many cases the outcome of an error in technology may not be observed for many years, and recent concern from a number of countries has highlighted the need for restraint in matters associated with xenotransplantation. Researchers and other scientists involved in producing transgenic organisms should be very aware of the welfare of transgenic animals and should strive to minimise the suffering of such animals, and in accordance with this requirement the Home Office has now drawn up additional rules to cover the welfare of and control of the distribution of transgenic species. These rules include a tight restriction on the suitability of rooms for holding and producing transgenic animals and the need for Home Office approval before transgenic species can be moved from one place to another.

Technically, human beings could be transformed using transgenic technology, although such experiments are, and should remain, illegal. Furthermore, there would be fears of unpredictable and perhaps irreversible side-effects that might occur in such individuals. It would be important to make the distinction between therapeutic and non-therapeutic genetic manipulations. Whereas therapeutic intervention aims to cure human disease, non-therapeutic therapy aims to influence some personal characteristic of the individual, e.g. to produce a child with increased intelligence, strength and/or height. In the Western world, it is not acceptable to choose the sex of a child purely on social grounds, although such a choice could be warranted if an individual was known to carry the gene for a serious sex-linked disorder that could result in the child inheriting the disease and dying in childhood. However, this only would be acceptable if an embryo was *selected* on the basis of not inheriting the disease rather than being genetically *manipulated*.

Conclusions and summary

At the present time, the costs and time involved in producing transgenic species are such that, apart from the development of various rodent models of human disease for research purposes, the technology is unlikely to become commonplace for some years. However, in some cases the creation of a transgenic animal for the purpose of producing a substance for human use, e.g. factor IX from sheep, is much cheaper than producing the same chemical in the laboratory (Concar, 1994). However, although an important consideration, cost should not be the prime factor in deciding whether to develop such models. It is as important to decide whether alternative methods are available and whether these are capable of producing a high-quality product in sufficient quantities for human use. The future potential of transgenic technology is such that it could conceivably produce models for numerous human diseases, thus enabling the mechanisms leading to the particular disease to be elucidated. In addition, these models would be suitable for determining the effectiveness of various therapeutic interventions. However, the consequences of this technology should be investigated and optimised fully before its use becomes widespread so that potential safety problems can be minimised, especially where xenograft procedures are involved.

References

Alberts B, Bray D, Lewis J, *et al.* (1989) Special features of plant cells. In: Alberts, B, *et al. Molecular Biology of the Cell*, 2nd edn. New York: Garland Publishing, pp 1137–1186.

Anon (1997) Cow's milk just like Mama makes. *New Scientist* 15 February, 12.

Barinaga M (1994) Knockout mice: round two. *Science* 265: 26–28.

Bramley P M (1997) Enhancing levels of carotenoids by genetic manipulation. *The Biochemist* 19: 16–20.

Breslow J L (1993) Transgenic mouse models of lipoprotein metabolism and atherosclerosis. *Proc Natl Acad Sci USA* 90: 8314–8318.

Brooks G (1994) Gene therapy. *Pharm J* 252: 256–260.

Brown P (1997) Pig transplants 'should be banned'. *New Scientist* 1 March, 6.

Casas A M, Kononowicz A K, Zehr U B, *et al.* (1993) Transgenic sorghum plants via microprojectile bombardment. *Proc Natl Acad Sci USA* 90: 11212–11216.

Coghlan A (1996) Gene trap catches 'knockout' mice. *New Scientist* 19 October, 22.

Concar D (1994) The organ factory of the future? *New Scientist* 18 June, 24–29.

Crabbe J C, Belknap J K, Buck K J (1994) Genetic animal models of alcohol and drug abuse. *Science* 264: 1715–1723.

Dorin J R, Dickinson P, Alton E W F W, *et al.* (1992) Cystic fibrosis in the mouse by targeted insertional mutagenesis. *Nature* 359: 211–215.

Field L J (1991) Cardiovascular research in transgenic animals. *Trends Cardiovasc Med* 1: 141–146.

Gurney M E, Pu H, Chiu A Y, *et al.* (1994) Motor neuron degeneration in mice that express a human Cu,Zn superoxide dismutase mutation. *Science* 264: 1772–1775.

Hogan B, Costantini F, Lacy E (eds) (1986) *Manipulating the Mouse Embryo. A Laboratory Manual.* Cold Spring Harbor, NY: Cold Spring Harbor Laboratory Press.

Isacson O, Breakefield X O (1997) Benefits and risks of hosting animal cells in the human brain. *Nature Med* 3: 964–969.

Jaenisch R (1977) Germ line integration of Moloney leukemia virus: effect of homozygosity at the m-mulV locus. *Cell* 12: 691–696.

Jaenisch R, Mintz B (1974) Simian virus 40 DNA sequences in DNA of healthy adult mice derived from preimplantation blastocysts injected with viral DNA. *Proc Natl Acad Sci USA* 71: 1250–1254.

Lawn R M, Wade D P, Hammer R E, *et al.* (1992) Atherogenesis in transgenic mice expressing human apolipoprotein(a). *Nature* 360: 670–672.

Mackenzie D (1996) Doctors farm fish for insulin. *New Scientist* 16 November, 20.

Mehtali M, Munschy M, Ali-Hadji D, Kieny M P (1992) A novel transgenic mouse model for the in vivo evaluation of anti-human immunodeficiency virus type 1 drugs. *Aids Research and Human Retroviruses* 8: 1959–1965.

Moore P (1993) Genetic manipulation. *New Scientist* (Inside Science No. 66), 1–4.

Ratcliff R, Evans M J, Cuthbert A W, *et al.* (1993) Production of a severe cystic fibrosis mutation in mice by gene targeting. *Nature Genet* 4: 35–41.

Williams N (1997) Pig–human transplants barred for now. *Science* 275: 473.

9

The use of peptides in the treatment of neurological disease

Sandra Amor

Advances in the production of synthetic peptides have allowed their use in both the laboratory setting as tools to examine biological responses and the development of novel therapeutic strategies for human diseases. This chapter will outline the importance of peptides in the maintenance of the nervous system and, conversely, their importance in inducing neurological diseases as a result of the induction of abnormal physiological responses. The induction of autoimmune responses to peptides ex-pressed within the central or peripheral nervous systems may ultimately lead to tissue damage and autoimmune disease. Deviation of the immune response with 'decoy' peptides and correction of abnormal physiological functions with 'normal' peptides has had some success in the experimental setting and will be discussed below. Finally, clinical trials in which peptides are used in therapeutic strategies in the treatment of the human neurological disorders Alzheimer's disease, myasthenia gravis and multiple sclerosis (MS) will be reviewed.

Proteins, peptides and amino acids

Diversity of proteins

The macromolecules that constitute cells can be classified into four categories: lipids, carbohydrates, nucleic acids and proteins. Proteins are the most complex and most abundant of the cellular components. The name protein (from the Greek *proteios* meaning 'of the first importance') was given to the substance extracted from plant and animal tissue by a Dutch chemist Gerardus Mulder in the nineteenth century that he believed to be the most important substance and without which life would not exist.

Proteins are diverse components and include enzymes, antibodies, hormones and cellular components such as myelin.

Composition of proteins

Proteins are composed of linear polymers termed polypeptides, which are formed from amino acids connected by peptide bonds. There are 20 amino acids, each with a core tetrahedral carbon atom covalently bonded to an amino group on one side and a carboxyl group on the other. The third bond is always hydrogen and the fourth is a variable side chain. There are various ways of classifying amino acids based on the variable side chain. The most common is the method of categorising amino acids according to the polarity of the amino acid, giving rise to eight relatively apolar amino acids, seven uncharged polar amino acids and five amino acids that exist in the uncharged state.

Amino acids are abbreviated by a three-letter or a single-letter code. An example of each group is represented by alanine (Ala; A), tyrosine (Tyr; Y) and lysine (Lys; K). Each amino acid may also be identified by its molecular weight, and thus the molecular weight of a chain of amino acids constituting a peptide may be determined.

Peptides

Peptides are formed by linking together the carboxyl end of one amino acid and the amino group of another. Any number of amino acids may be joined successively to form a peptide chain. Thus, at one end of the peptide/protein is the the free amino group, i.e. the amino- or N-terminal end, while at the other, carboxy-terminal or C-terminal, end is the free carboxyl group. A small protein may be composed of only 50 amino acids, whereas longer ones may be composed of 3000 or more. For example, in the myelin sheath, the major myelin component, myelin basic protein, is composed of 166 amino acids and proteolipid protein of 271 amino acids.

However, a native protein is not purely a string of amino acids. Additional modification of the protein chain is made following translation of the sequence during protein synthesis in the cell. As a rule, central nervous system (CNS) myelin proteins are covalently modified following their biosynthesis. Glycosylation, acylation, acetylation, methylation, deamidation, deimination and phosphorylation are among the common modifications that CNS myelin proteins undergo. Patterns of such modification change as the individual develops or as damage or stress occurs and tissue regeneration takes place. It is possible that altered myelin determinants play a role in the development or perpetuation of autoimmune responses in MS and other nervous system diseases.

Production of synthetic peptides

Each peptide and protein is uniquely characterised by its amino acid composition and sequence. To determine the sequence, it is necessary to break the chain, separate the amino acids and determine the relative quantities of each amino acid. The sequence may be determined by various chemical reactions and is ultimately dependent on the type of amino acid found at the end of each fragment.

Similarly, knowledge of the biochemistry of proteins and peptides has prompted the development of techniques for synthesising peptides with predetermined sequences, such as myelin basic protein and proteolipid protein. In neurological research, synthesis of peptides and polypeptides has been invaluable for the study of the pathogenic processes in disease and in the development of novel therapeutic strategies (Chapter 11).

To synthesise a peptide in the laboratory, several biochemical problems need to be overcome. To produce a set sequence it is essential that the amino group of one amino acid is linked to the carboxyl group of another and not to itself or to the side chains of another amino acid. Thus, such undesired linkages must be blocked or prevented. The next step is to allow the unprotected carboxyl group to be activated and the two amino acids coupled together. The final step is to remove the blocking agent. The most popular method is called the Merrifield process, which involves attaching the C-terminal amino acid to a resin. Manual production has largely been superseded by automated peptide synthesisers, which, although expensive, are able to make milligram and gram quantities of multiple peptides sequences within hours. The purity of the peptide is controlled by high-performance liquid chromatography (HPLC) and the quality of peptide assessed by mass spectrometry based on the known molecular weight of the peptide of choice.

Such technology also allows the synthesis of modified peptides (addition of native post-translational modifications) more akin to the native sequence, which may be important in some biochemical and immunological reactions.

Uses of synthetic peptides

Purified native proteins have the obvious advantage of being in a more natural state than synthetically produced compounds. However, in the case of proteins that exist in very small quantities in the native state, a complicated and expensive procedure is necessary to produce significant quantities for study. Thus synthetic proteins, produced by molecular biological techniques of cloning specific genes into vectors and the production of recombinant proteins, have become popular. In addition, advances in chemical procedures mean that the production of synthetic peptides for many aspects of scientific research and therapies is becoming less expensive and more popular.

Some areas making use of synthetic peptides include:

1   monoclonal antibody production (Chapter 11);
2   screening patients for serum reactivity to known peptides using immunoassays;
3   vaccination;
4   therapeutic strategies in experimental and human diseases.

Immune responses to peptides

To understand how peptides may be used to control neurological diseases such as those thought to be due to an autoimmune response, e.g. multiple sclerosis, it is first necessary to explain how the immune response responds to peptides and how such diseases may arise. For more information the reader is referred to Janeway and Travers (1996). Understanding how the immune response causes tissue damage has allowed the development of strategies in which the immune response can be modulated using 'decoy' peptides.

Immune responses in infections

An immune response is initiated to defend the host against invading micro-organisms (antigens). Such infection results in a cascade of events to rid the host of the pathogen, including activation of cells such as macrophages and lymphocytes. While some of these cells phagocytose the organism (i.e. macrophages), other cells secrete antibodies (i.e. B lymphocytes) as well as produce chemicals (e.g. cytokines and free oxygen radicals), which may themselves be toxic or may augment the immune response, making it more efficient to deal with the infection.

Immune responses to self antigens

The immune response is also important in non-infectious situations such as allergies and autoimmune diseases in which the response is directed to self antigens. Immune responses are also important in rejection of transplanted organs and tissue grafts, and immunologists are attempting to control these immunological reactions, which cause rather than prevent disease.

Activation of T cells

A lymphocyte is activated when its receptor on the cell surface binds to an antigen. It is thought that, during development, lymphocytes that encounter self antigens are eliminated and are thus self-tolerant. However, this may not always be the case, as responses to self tissue, which may lead to autoimmune disease, sometimes occur.

When a micro-organism enters the host, each activated lymphocyte gives rise to progeny with the same receptor and then to effector cells which, for example, secrete antibody. For example, T lymphocytes when activated become 'killer cells', which eliminate other cells infected with micro-organisms, or become so-called 'helper cells', which activate other cells of the immune system, including macrophages and B lymphocytes, that produce antibodies.

Activation of all T cells involves the recognition of peptide fragments of antigens bound to cell-surface proteins called major histocompatability complex (MHC) molecules. The type of MHC molecules found on T cells varies between individuals, and peptide fragments that fit into one type of MHC molecule and activate one person's T cells may be unable to fit into another person's MHC molecule and thus be unable to activate that individual's T cells. The MHC in humans is a polymorphic cluster of genes and is of extreme interest to immunologists because the polymorphism may explain susceptibility to many immunological disorders, including autoimmune diseases.

Antigen processing

T cells are able to respond to peptide antigens, whether viral or self antigens, displayed on the cell surface in the MHC molecules. For peptide fragments to be associated with the MHC molecule, the protein must first be degraded inside the cell and carried to the cell surface by the MHC molecules. The type of antigen encountered will determine not only how the peptide is processed, but also the type of MHC molecule used, the phenotype of the lymphocyte and its effector function. Thus, in the case of cytosolic pathogens such as viruses, the degradation process occurs in the cytoplasm and peptides bind to MHC class I molecules. These are able to activate CD8 T cells, resulting in death of the infected cell. Alternatively, extracellular pathogens and antigens (such as self antigens) are degraded in acidified vesicles and then presented in association with MHC class II molecules, which activate CD4 lymphocytes.

Presentation of peptides

MHC molecules are glycoproteins, the structures of which have been determined by X-ray crystallography. The MHC class II molecule is composed of two transmembrane chains: α and β. Together these form a structure containing a cleft in which the 'floor' is made by the β-sheets and the sides by the α-helices (Figure 9.1). The peptide is bound within the cleft.

Pockets within the MHC molecule allow amino acids from the

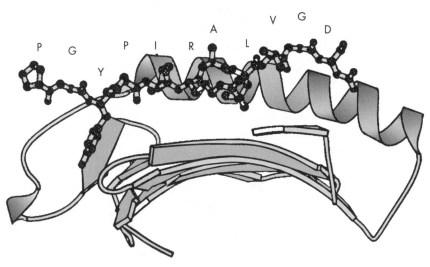

Figure 9.1 Diagrammatic representation of MHC–peptide interactions predicted by computer modelling. The side view of the MHC class II molecule of Biozzi ABH mice (H-2A^{g7}) is represented as a ribbon. Within the cleft of the class II molecule lies the peptide sequence PGYPIRALVGD (ball and stick) of myelin oligodendrocyte glycoprotein (MOG), which induces the experimental autoimmune model of multiple sclerosis.

peptide fragment to interact with the amino acids of the MHC and anchor the peptide. The strength and type of interaction depends on the nature of the amino acids in the peptide and those of the MHC molecules that line the pockets. Some peptide amino acids are more important in binding and are called anchor residues. Several studies have demonstrated the importance of these anchor residues, as changing any of the anchor residues prevents the peptide binding. Altering amino acid residues may also change the binding affinity of the peptides, causing them to bind more or less strongly, as well as changing how the T cell recognises the peptide.

Activation of T cells

T-cell receptors (TCRs) resemble immunoglobulin molecules (Chapter 11). They are heterodimers which, like the MHC molecule, are composed of two transmembrane glycoprotein chains: α and β. The TCR is anchored in the membrane of the cell, and a short segment connects the immunoglobulin-like domains to the membrane (the hinge region). The immunoglobulin-like domains are composed of a constant region (C) and a variable region (V). Although recognition of peptide in the context of MHC molecules occurs via the V region of the TCR (Figure 9.2), activation also requires other co-stimulatory signals, although these will not be discussed here.

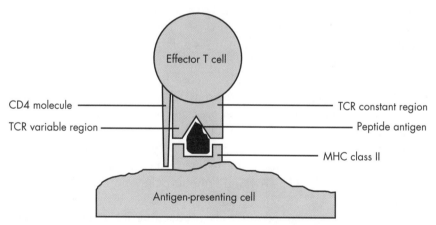

Figure 9.2 Diagrammatic representation of T-cell–peptide–MHC interaction. The MHC class II molecule expressed on antigen-presenting cells presents the peptide antigen to the TCR. The variable region of the TCR recognises the peptide in context with MHC class II and becomes activated.

Activation of T cells changes a number of cell-surface molecules and induces the release of chemicals called cytokines. Some of the cell-surface molecules allow the T lymphocytes entry to sites of inflammation, which ensures that they are able to circulate through tissue to encounter and remove antigen. These molecules are called cell adhesion molecules, i.e. they allow the cell to 'adhere' to the endothelial cell and cross into the tissue. One such adhesion molecule is VLA-4, which binds to other adhesion molecules on the endothelial cell. VLA-4 also binds to an extracellular matrix protein, fibronectin, specifically at a region of the protein termed CS-1. Of interest is the finding that blocking this adhesion molecule with monoclonal antibodies to VLA-4 inhibits the induction of an experimental model of multiple sclerosis. Furthermore, synthetic peptides corresponding to peptides of the CS-1 protein of fibronectin are also able to block VLA-4 activity, although to date these studies have been restricted to inflammatory disease and these findings have not been demonstrated in neurological disease.

Cytokines

Once activated, T cells may perform a number of effector and signalling functions, including the activation of other effector cells in the immune system, such as cytotoxic T cells, macrophages and B cells, via direct cell-to-cell contact or by secretion of a large array of signalling molecules, including cytokines. Soluble factors such as cytokines are critically involved in determining which functions will be developed to an effector stage and which functions will remain silent. It is accepted that production of certain types of cytokines produced by activated T cells may be classified in two major groups. Those that promote the inflammatory processes, cell-mediated immune responses and less pronounced antibody formation are usually called type 1 helper cells (Th1 cells) and the response they provoke is referred to as the type 1 response. The major cytokines that belong to this group are interferon gamma (IFN-γ), tumour necrosis factor alpha (TNF-α) and lymphotoxin, and these T cells also produce interleukin 2 (IL-2). The other group is associated with immune responses involving marked antibody production, including IgG2b, IgE and IgA, with less inflammation, and their response is generally referred to as a type 2 response. Accordingly, T cells that are involved in the development of such a response are termed type 2 helper (Th2) cells. Prime cytokines belonging to this group are IL-4, IL-5 and IL-10. Although in most cases mature, activated T cells produce cytokines that are representatives of just one of the two groups, this dichotomy is not absolute and hybrid production of both type 1 and type 2 cytokines by a single T cell is not a very unusual event. Based on experiences in studies of mucosal immune responses, some investigators have suggested the existence of a third type of T cell, tentatively designated Th3, that is characterised by secretion of transforming growth factor beta (TGF-β). This cytokine has peculiar, broad suppressive effects in a large array of immune effector systems. This proposal is, however, still controversial and requires further substantiation. In a more general sense, cytokines belonging to either type 1 or type 2 immune responses will favour the maturation and activation of other T cells with the same type of effector function, in this way amplifying the immune response while keeping its quality the same.

Why particular T cells are selected to be Th1 or Th2 type is unknown, but the quality and affinity of TCR interaction with peptide in context with MHC may be an important factor.

The nervous system

The nervous system is divided into the peripheral nervous system (PNS) and CNS. For the purpose of this review, the major cell types of the CNS and PNS will be outlined and where appropriate those involved in neurological diseases mentioned.

Nerves, axons, oligodendrocytes and myelin

The CNS receives information from the sensory organs via the PNS: the nervous impulses are transmitted along axons, which are protected by myelin. In Alzheimer's disease atrophy, degeneration and the presence of neuro-fibrillary changes in nerve cells give rise to dementia. In some severe cases disintegration of the tissue may be so complete that few nerve cells are observed.

In the CNS, the myelin is produced by oligodendrocytes, whereas that in the PNS is produced by Schwann cells. Demyelination (breakdown of myelin) is associated with an impaired conductivity, which leads to a variety of neurological signs and symptoms. Several demyelinating diseases of both the PNS, e.g. Guillain–Barré syndrome, and the CNS, e.g. multiple sclerosis and subacute sclerosis panencephalitis, are known. Demyelination is also observed in neuro-AIDS.

In some of these diseases, myelin damage may be the result of an autoimmune response whereby the immune system is activated by myelin components. Mechanisms by which the inflammatory, tissue-damaging immune response is either switched off or diverted to a non-inflammatory state is a major research topic not only in the area of neurological research but also in the study of many other diseases such as rheumatoid arthritis, uveitis and diabetes. As discussed above, the type of immune response, i.e. proinflammatory (Th1) or regulatory (Th2), depends on the type of peptide–MHC interaction and thus current studies are using peptides in the development of novel therapies in these diseases.

Autoimmune diseases of the neuromuscular junction are relatively uncommon and are sometimes associated with other autoimmune diseases. In myasthenia gravis, there is degeneration of the post-synaptic regions of the motor endplate and a deficiency of acetylcholine receptors at the endplate.

Myelin proteins

Myelin sheaths are composed of 75–80% lipids and 20–25% proteins. The two most abundant proteins in myelin are the hydrophobic transmembrane protein proteolipid protein (PLP), which accounts for about 50% of the total protein in myelin, and the strongly hydrophilic myelin basic protein (MBP), which makes up 10–15% of all protein. In addition to these abundant proteins, myriad other proteins are found associated with CNS myelin, each of which usually does not represent more than 1% of the total protein mass. These include structural proteins such as myelin-associated glycoprotein (MAG) and myelin oligodendrocyte glycoprotein (MOG), which have a role in the maintenance of the myelin structure and its interactions with other cellular components as well as enzymes such as CNPase, transaldolase-H, kinases, acyltransferases and methylases that can modify the myelin structure upon receiving the appropriate signals. Glycosylation, acylation, acetylation, methylation, deamidation, deimination and phosphorylation are among the common modifications that CNS myelin proteins undergo. Patterns of such modification change as the individual develops or as damage or stress occurs and tissue regeneration takes place.

Neurological diseases

Alzheimer's disease

Alzheimer's disease is a chronic dementia and neurodegenerative disorder affecting a large percentage of the population. Large quantities of a peptide derived from amyloid precursor protein (β-APP) are found in plaques within the brains of these patients and are thought to be the principal cause of cell damage. The β-APP peptide 1–40 is able to form abnormal channels in lipid bilayers. It may therefore be possible to target this peptide for therapy in this disease.

Guillain–Barré syndrome

Guillain–Barré syndrome (GBS) is an acute demyelinating polyneuropathy of unknown aetiology and pathogenesis. A role for autoimmunity is suggested by the findings that affected patients have antibodies and T cells directed at myelin components of the PNS. Furthermore, the clinical course of GBS correlates with titres of antibodies to peripheral nerve myelin and antibodies.

Experimental allergic neuritis

Experimental GBS may be induced in animals with peripheral myelin and peptide fragments of myelin proteins. This experimental model disease is called experimental allergic neuritis (EAN) and is induced in Lewis rats with the peripheral nervous myelin protein P2-derived sequence 53–78.

Myasthenia gravis

The prevalence of myasthenia gravis is approximately 5–7.5/100 000. The disease is first observed as muscle weakness which gradually progresses throughout the body. The disease most likely results from the presence of antibodies directed against the acetylcholine receptor (AchR). Genetic studies have shown that both susceptibility and resistance to myasthenia gravis is influenced by HLA (tissue) type (McCombe, 1995) and there is also an association with immunoglobulin isotypes. Histologically the disease manifests itself by degeneration of the post-synaptic regions of the motor endplate. Although there are no signs of inflammation in these regions, perivascular infiltrates are observed in the muscle.

Experimental myasthenia gravis

Experimental allergic myasthenia gravis can be induced in rodents following the passive transfer of anti-AchR antibodies, following immunisation with recombinant AchR subunit administered in adjuvants or by passive transfer of AchR-sensitised lymphocytes. This strongly suggests that, at least in this case, T cells are somehow involved. Lewis rats immunised with either a subunit of AchR or the peptide sequence 100–116 exhibit disease.

Multiple sclerosis

Multiple sclerosis (MS) is an inflammatory and demyelinating disease of the CNS. Epidemiological studies have demonstrated that the disease affects 5–300 per 100 000 people in Western societies, although there are high-, medium- and low-risk areas. The aetiology of the disease is unknown, although many viruses have been implicated in the onset and progression of the disease (Russell, 1997). Once initiated, however, the disease is probably autoimmune mediated. The idea that immune mechanisms are important in MS is supported by the finding that T and B cells respond to myelin antigens such as MBP, PLP, MOG, MAG and other antigens, e.g. the heat shock protein alpha B-crystallin (Van Noort *et al.*, 1995).

Experimental allergic encephalomyelitis

A role for autoimmunity in multiple sclerosis is also supported by data from the experimental autoimmune model experimental allergic encephalomyelitis (EAE), which may be induced by CNS antigens in rodents and primates. Immunisation of animals with spinal cord homogenate induces EAE (Figure 9.3), as does immunisation with individual myelin proteins or peptides of these antigens. Chronic-relapsing EAE is more reminiscent of MS because animals develop accumulating neurological deficits and demyelination following each disease phase. In mice, the onset of disease is observed as a weight loss followed by increasing neurological deficit (Amor *et al.*, 1994).

Experimental allergic encephalomyelitis may be induced with whole myelin, e.g. homogenates of spinal cord tissue from naive animals, or with purified preparations of myelin proteins isolated from the homogenate. However, as discussed above, it may be difficult to isolate sufficient quantities of protein for study, and researchers have turned to molecular biological methods of making recombinant proteins or using synthetic peptides. In this way, a number of myelin proteins that can induce EAE in different animals have been identified. In particular, the

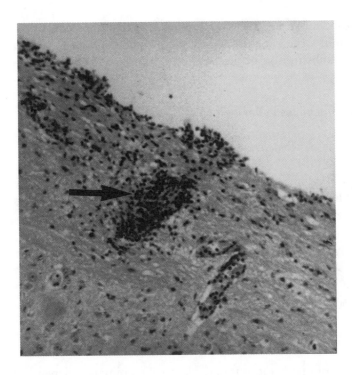

Figure 9.3 Inflammation of the spinal cord of a Biozzi ABH mouse during the acute clinical phase of chronic-relapsing experimental autoimmune encephalomyelitis following injection with spinal cord homogenate and adjuvant.

Table 9.1 Peptide sequence of myelin protein able to induce EAE in mice expressing particular class II molecules

Mouse strain	MHC class II	Myelin protein and peptide sequence		
		MBP	MOG	PLP
Biozzi ABH	g7	12–26	8–22	56–70
SJL	s	89–101	92–106	139–151
PLJ	u	Ac1–11	35–55	43–64G

use of inbred mice and rats has identified specific fragments of the protein that are encephalitogenic, i.e. induce disease (Table 9.1).

Characterisation of encephalitogenic epitopes of myelin antigens has enabled studies at the molecular level of peptide–MHC and peptide–MHC–T cell receptor interactions that are relevant to disease. Furthermore, the anchor residues for specific peptides have been examined and substitution of these residues found to alter disease.

The use of peptides in the therapy of neurological diseases

Therapies in autoimmune neurological diseases

Therapies for autoimmune diseases have focused on two strategies for re-establishment of immunological tolerance. The first involves changing an antigen-specific response from a proinflammatory response into a regulatory response. In this context, tolerance means not a lack of responsiveness but rather a lack of pathogenic responsiveness. The second strategy involves deletion or inactivation of antigen-specific T cells, i.e. developing ways to kill autoreactive T cells by the induction of apoptosis.

Routes of administration

Induction of many autoimmune diseases in animals is dependent on the injection of adjuvants (substances that enhance the response) together with the antigens and the route of administration. Intraperitoneal, subcutaneous and intradermal routes are effective, whereas administration of antigens via the oral or intranasal route is not. It seems that the way in which the immune system deals with antigens that enter the body via the nasal or oral mucosa or via the gastrointestinal tract is different from what happens during classical immunisation. Instead of activating T cells capable of secreting IFN-γ, lymphotoxin or TNF-α (type 1 responses), oral administration appears to activate T cells that secrete large amounts of TGF-β, a modulatory cytokine (Miller *et al.*, 1993). Such T cells, tentatively designated Th3 cells, may down-regulate inflammatory responses and, at least in experimental models, they ameliorate autoimmune responses (Weiner *et al.*, 1994). In this way, oral or intranasal administration of MBP modulates EAE in rats.

Ongoing clinical trials in MS are based on the expectation that, by oral administration of the putative autoantigen(s) (i.e. a myelin protein), it may be possible to shift the specific immune response to one that is less inflammatory. However, this approach may not be as straightforward as one would hope. First, steering the autoantigen-directed response in patients suffering from, for example, MS to type 2 responses may not be helpful if pathogenic antibodies are implicated in the disease. Also, oral administration of antigen may very well lead to activation of some pathogenic T cells, including cytotoxic T cells, as was recently found in marmosets (Genain et al., 1996) as well as in mice. Thus, many questions still remain to be answered regarding the exact way in which the immune system deals with orally or intranasally administered antigen and what the final outcome of this strategy might be. The ability to control inflammatory responses in this way is sufficiently provocative and useful to justify ongoing efforts to try and find the appropriate answers.

A different mechanism involved in the re-establishment of tolerance is co-stimulation or, rather, the lack of co-stimulation. As explained above, T cells encounter their antigen in the context of MHC molecules; however, they die in the absence of the necessary co-stimulatory molecules. Thus, therapies should be aimed at the administration of antigen that T cells would encounter in the context of MHC molecules but in the absence of co-stimulation. Experimental approaches to achieve this include oral administration of antigen, intravenous administration of antigen, intraperitoneal administration in incomplete adjuvant or administration of chemically prepared peptide–antigen–MHC complexes. In all cases, co-stimulation does not occur and T cells reactive to the introduced antigen undergo apoptotic death. In experimental models of autoimmunity, this approach has been quite successful both with proteins and with peptides.

Experimental allergic encephalomyelitis

Altered peptide ligands

As discussed above, T-cell activation occurs when the TCR engages with the MHC molecule in which a specific peptide is bound. Identification of autoantigenic peptides such as the encephalitogenic peptides MOG, PLP and MBP, which induce EAE in mice such as the Biozzi ABH mouse (Amor et al., 1993), and studies on how they interact with MHC class II molecules and the TCR have allowed the development of altered peptide ligands (APLs), i.e. altered peptide sequences of PLP, MBP and MOG. Thus, in the Biozzi ABH mouse, although the PLP 56–70 sequence DYEYLINVIHAFQYV induces chronic-relapsing EAE, an APL in which the histidine (H) at position 65 is replaced by a lysine (K) does not induce disease. Subtle changes in the sequence of APL compared with the wild-type peptide may alter the affinity of binding to the MHC. Alternatively, such changes may occur in the regions of the peptide recognised by the TCR. Thus, the APL may result in a different cell response from that induced by the original peptide. In this way APLs have been shown to inhibit (antagonise) or augment (superagonise) the normal T-cell response, while others are able to deviate (partially agonise) the response completely, e.g. changing a Th1 response to a Th2 response.

In the PLJ mouse EAE model, the MBP peptide Ac1–11 (Ac ASQKRPSQRSK) is the immunodominant epitope for induction of disease. The amino acids important in MHC binding and those thought to be the major T-cell contact points have been identified. Computer modelling using the crystal structure of an MHC molecule can be used to evaluate possible ways in which a short peptide sequence may interact with the peptide-binding cleft of the MHC molecule. In the case of the MBP sequence binding to the MHC class II molecule of the PLJ mouse, substitution at position 4 results in peptides with different affinities for the MHC. It is striking that the original encephalitogenic epitope binds with only low affinity. This low-affinity binding has been suggested to be a major reason why potentially responsive T cells may escape negative selection in the thymus (reviewed by Fairchild and Wraith, 1996). In another model of EAE, the SJL mouse, the major immunodominant epitope is the PLP sequence 139–151 (HSLGKWLGHPDKF). Adoptive transfer of Th1 CD4+ lymphocyte clones against this sequence induces disease in recipient mice. Generation of T-cell clones has shown that Th1-like cells are able to induce disease, and the major TCR binding sites for Th1 cells are W at position 144 and H at position 147 (Kuchroo et al., 1994). Likewise, the MHC contact points have been identified as L at position 145 and P at position 148. The use of peptide analogues has demonstrated that tryptophan (W) at position 144 is critical for TCR contact and activation. Substitution of glutamine (Q) for tryptophan (W) (HSLGKQLGHPDKF) abolishes the ability of the peptide to induce disease, suggesting that peptide analogues may exert their activity via competition with the wild type owing to the higher binding affinity of the analogues for MHC. The T cells induced by the APLs produced a predominantly type 2 response (IL-10, IL-4), demonstrating that APLs were able to skew the cytokine profile. In protection studies, co-immunisation of the authentic peptide with the glutamine APL protects mice from EAE. Furthermore, an analogue peptide with leucine at position 144 and arginine at 147 does not cause EAE but can prevent disease induction. However, the mechanism by which APLs exert their effect has not been fully elucidated. It is probable that T-cell manipulation by APLs is based on the differential activation of selected intracellular signalling pathways.

Soluble MHC class II–peptide complexes

In SJL mice, the immunodominant MBP peptide sequence 91–103 induces EAE – the autoimmune model of MS. These mice express the particular class II molecule referred to as I-A^s. Injection of a formulation in which soluble MHC molecules are associated with the peptide 91–103 has been found to halt the progression of EAE in mice.

Copolymer 1

Copolymer 1 (Copaxone®) is a synthetic amino acid copolymer of L-alanine, L-glutamic acid, L-lysine and L-tyrosine and cross-reacts with MBP. Intradermal injection of Copolymer 1 prevents EAE in the guinea pig prior to the onset of disease and at the time of clinical onset. The mode of action is thought to be the generation of suppressor T cells and inhibition of MBP-reactive T cells.

Targeting the TCR

Many experimental studies in EAE have demonstrated that the pathogenic (encephalitogenic) T cells are highly restricted in their V structures, all sharing more or less the same structure. Thus, therapies designed to block autoimmunity by intervening at the level of TCRs were developed. These included the administration of Vβ-specific antibodies, immunisation with peptides representing the V sequence in order to induce regulatory immunity against pathogenic T cells and whole T-cell vaccination. Many of these therapies were quite successful in blocking the development of EAE.

Research evolved to also include studies on Vβ sequences and the CDR3 junctional region of TCR sequences. Vandenbark *et al.* (1996) demonstrated that immunisation with the synthetic peptide (39–59) representing the hypervariable region of the Vβ8 molecule protected Lewis rats against EAE. Immunisation with this peptide also induced antibodies directed against Vβ8 which could also protect against disease. Protection was also attributed to regulatory T cells directed to the TCR.

Thus, the results of studies examining therapies targeting the TCR suggest that peptide therapy maybe be useful in human disease.

Experimental allergic neuritis

EAN, as described above, may be induced by co-administration of neuro-antigen and adjuvants. It is well known that interactions occur between the immune, nervous and endocrine systems. This is classically demonstrated in adrenalectomised animals, in which stressful events have been shown to modulate autoimmune disease. In the EAN model of GBS, the peptide ACTH-9 analogue, which does not exhibit corticotrophic or melanotrophic action, has been shown to modulate disease. Furthermore, histological examination has demonstrated complete preservation of myelinated nerves, suggesting that neuropeptide treatment may be useful in the clinical setting although the exact mechanism of action remains to be determined.

Experimental allergic myasthenia gravis

Soluble MHC class II–peptide complexes

Experimental allergic myasthenia gravis may be induced by co-administration of AchR and adjuvant. In rats the immunodominant epitope 100–116 also induces disease. Intravenous injection of soluble MHC purified from rats and coupled to the peptide 100–116 reduces T-cell proliferative responses in these animals and increases the survival of these animals.

Alzheimer's disease

The precursor protein beta/4A (APP) is involved in the regulation of neural growth and survival and has recently been shown to be neurotrophic (Bowes et al., 1994), suggesting that therapy with this peptide may be useful to overcome neurodegeneration. Bowes et al. further demonstrated that the tropic properties were contained within a short sequence of the protein, i.e. a 17 amino acid peptide. In rabbits, this peptide was able to attenuate neuronal dysfunction or loss and behaviour deficits associated with neuronal injury. The peptide was effective when administered intrathecally 20 minutes before and daily ($\times$3) after ischaemia was induced in the spinal cord.

Problems with peptide therapies

Thus, at least in experimental animals, peptide therapy of neurological diseases has been shown to be successful. Some of these therapies are now in clinical trials and the results obtained so far suggest that peptide therapies may be applicable in other diseases. However, in many cases, this assumes that the peptides administered are not themselves pathogenic and that in diseases in which multiple antigens are likely to be involved such specific therapy with a single peptide is effective.

Clinical trials

Soluble MHC class II–peptide complexes

Multiple sclerosis

In patients with MS, the major class II molecule associated with disease is the HLA-DR2 molecule. Although the peptides that induce disease cannot be determined, the immunodominant T-cell epitopes have been suggested by *in vitro* immunological methods. Thus, for MBP the epitope 84–102 has been shown to be the immunodominant epitope and has been used in conjunction with MHC class II molecules to suppress T-cell proliferation *in vitro*.

For DRβ1*1501 – a subtype of the DR2 MHC molecule – the peptide motif that binds to this MHC molecule has been shown to be MBP 84–102, amino acid sequence DENP<u>VVHFFKNIV</u>TPRTPP (the core sequence is underlined).

A T-cell clone from a patient expressing DRβ1*1501 proliferates extensively in the presence of this peptide and macrophages, i.e. cells that present this peptide to the TCR and induce T-cell activation. However, the MHC–peptide (DR2–MBP84–102) complex significantly reduces this T-cell activity. This reduction in activity is associated with altered cytokine secretion. Phase I and phase II trials of the drug Anergen in relapsing remitting MS are in progress in the USA.

Myasthenia gravis

In myasthenia gravis patients, a haplotype particularly associated with disease is DR4 Dw14.2 and the peptide is AchR 144–163. The sequence of this peptide is MKLGT<u>WTYDGSVV</u>AINPESD (the core sequence is underlined). Again, proliferation of patients' T cells occurs vigorously in the presence of peptide and macrophages but not if the peptide is applied in combination with soluble MHC molecules. Again, such antigen-specific therapy offers a rational approach to the immunotherapy of autoimmune diseases.

TCR peptides

Pathogenic T cells can be distinguished from all other T cells by their TCRs, and for many experimental autoimmune diseases the major T-cell sequence in disease induction is Vβ8.2, although there are exceptions. Thus, T cells expressing this Vβ sequence have been targeted in therapies in humans with autoimmune diseases.

Multiple sclerosis

The use of TCR peptides has been applied to the treatment of MS patients. Initially analysis of TCR Vβ in MS patients revealed the dominant Vβ epitopes to be Vβ6, Vβ5 and Vβ2. In a phase I trial, the optimal dose was found to be two intramuscular injections 4 weeks apart. Therapy reduced the number of Vβ6 cells in the cerebrospinal fluid. A further trial with a peptide of Vβ5 was also reported (Vandenbark *et al.*, 1996). In this study, a TCR peptide vaccine developed from the Vβ5 sequence that is expressed in MS plaques and on MBP-specific T cells was found to increase the number of peptide-reactive T cells in patients with progressive MS. Vaccine responders had a reduced MBP response and remained clinically stable after one year, whereas non-responders had an increased MBP response and progressed clinically. Peptide-specific Th2 cells directly inhibited MBP-specific T helper 1 cells *in vitro* through the release of IL-10, implicating a bystander suppression mechanism of action. The Vβ5 peptide phase I trial is being carried out by Connective Therapeutics in the USA.

Altered peptide ligands

The use of an APL with MBP antagonist properties has been studied in a phase I trial in 30 patients in the USA and Canada – the data have not yet been reported.

Copolymer 1

Copolymer 1 (Copaxone®) is a synthetic amino acid copolymer. It is able in a variety of species to suppress EAE induced by injection of spinal cord homogenate or purified MBP and PLP. The sequence of copolymer 1 is reported to be very similar to the immunodominant epitope of MBP and there is a marked degree of immunological cross-reactivity in both the cellular and humoral responses between MBP and copolymer 1. In the clinical setting, in a US phase III trial the following effects were observed in MS patients:

1   reduction in relapse rate of 32%;
2   an increase in the number of relapse-free patients;
3   fewer relapses per patient;
4   patients improved on copolymer 1 compared with placebo ($P = 0.02$).

Although the mechanism of action is unknown, from experimental study it has been postulated that the peptide either competes at the MHC level with peptides that induce disease or induces antigen-specific suppressor T cells (Arnon *et al.*, 1996). The peptide was approved by the FDA for relapsing remitting MS in December 1996, launched in the USA in January 1997 and should be available in the UK in the near future.

Conclusions

The use of specific peptide therapies in neurological diseases such as those discussed above has the advantage compared with non-specific therapies, such as immunosuppressant drugs, that not all the host's immune responses are inhibited. Delineating patterns of antigen reactivity as a function of disease duration or disease activity are clearly important for the design of therapeutic strategies. For diseases such as myasthenia gravis and multiple sclerosis, experimental data have now allowed experimental therapies to move to the clinic and should lend hope to other patients with neurological diseases in which peptides may play a role in the pathogenesis.

Acknowledgments

The author's research is supported by the Multiple Sclerosis Society of Great Britain and Northern Ireland and the European Commission via the T-cell autoimmunity in MS Concerted Action Programme.

References

Amor S, Baker D, Groome N, *et al.* (1993) Identification of a major encephalitogenic epitope of proteolipid protein (residues 56–70) for the induction of experimental allergic encephalomyelitis in Biozzi AB/H and non-obese diabetic mice. *J Immunol* 150: 5666–5672.

Amor S, Groome N, Linington C, *et al.* (1994) Identification of epitopes of myelin oligodendrocyte glycoprotein for the induction of experimental allergic encephalomyelitis in SJL and Biozzi AB/H mice. *J Immunol* 153: 4349–4356.

Arnon R, Sela M, Teitelbaum D (1996) New insights into the mechanism of action of copolymer 1 in experimental allergic encephalomyelitis and multiple sclerosis. *J Neurol* 243: 8–13.

Bowes M P, Masliah E, Otero D A, *et al.* (1994) Reduction of neurological damage by a peptide segment of the amyloid beta/A4 protein precursor in a rabbit spinal cord ischemia model. *Exp Neurol* 129: 112–119.

Fairchild P J, Wraith D C (1996) Lowering the tone: mechanisms of immunodominance among epitopes with low affinity for MHC. *Immunol Today* 17: 80–85.

Genain C P, Abel K, Belmar N, *et al.* (1996) Late complications of immune deviation therapy in a nonhuman primate. *Science* 274: 2054–2057.

Janeway C A, Travers P, eds. (1996) *Immunobiology*, 2nd edn. Oxford: Blackwell Scientific Publications.

Kuchroo V K, Greer J M, Kaul D, *et al.* (1994) A single TCR antagonist peptide inhibits allergic encephalomyelitis mediated by a diverse T cell repertoire. *J Immunol* 153: 3326–3336.

McCombe P A (1995) Autoimmune diseases of the neuromuscular junction and other disorders of the motor unit. In: Pender M P, McCombe P A, eds. *Autoimmune Neurological Disease*. Cambridge: Cambridge University Press, pp 257–330.

Miller A, al-Sabbagh A, Santos L M B, *et al.* (1993) Epitopes of myelin basic protein that trigger TGF-β release after oral tolerization are distinct from encephalitogenic epitopes and mediate epitope-driven bystander suppression. *J Immunol* 151: 7307–7315.

Russell W C (1997) Viruses and MS. In: Russell W C, ed. *Molecular Biology of Multiple Sclerosis*. Chichester: John Wiley, pp 243–254.

Vandenbark A A, Chou Y K, Whitham R, *et al.* (1996) Treatment of multiple sclerosis with T-cell receptor peptides: results of a double-blind pilot trial. *Nat Med* 2: 1109–1115.

Van Noort J M, van Sechel A C, Bajramovic J J, *et al.* (1995) The small heat-shock protein αβ-crystallin as candidate autoantigen in multiple sclerosis. *Nature* 375: 798–801.

Weiner H L, Friedman A, Miller A, *et al.* (1994) Oral tolerance: immunologic mechanisms and treatment of animal and human organ-specific autoimmune disease by oral administration of autoantigens. *Annu Rev Immunol* 12: 809–837.

10

Cytokines in cancer treatment

Vanessa Potter and Penella J Woll

Throughout the twentieth century, physicians have sought to harness the natural defences of the human body to fight cancer. William B Coley (1862–1936) was an early enthusiast for this approach. This New York City surgeon had observed spontaneous regression of tumours in some patients with severe bacterial infections and he started experimenting with the use of bacterial culture filtrates to treat cancers. Patients treated with 'Coley's toxin' frequently experienced fevers, rigors and other unpleasant side-effects, but occasional successes were achieved. Coley's experience exemplifies the difficulty of studying the effects of cytokines. Although the natural compounds are present in very small amounts and are difficult to isolate, the availability of recombinant proteins has revolutionised progress in the past 25 years. Their actions have, however, been difficult to define because the cytokines typically act in concert and their effects are mediated by the release of a cascade of intermediaries. It now appears that Coley's toxin was a bacterial lipopolysaccharide endotoxin that is a potent stimulus for the release of host cytokines, including interferons, interleukins and tumour necrosis factor.

Cytokines have proved difficult to evaluate in the same way as conventional pharmacological agents. Unlike most drugs, they are proteins whose actions are mediated by specific high-affinity cell-surface receptors. The resultant cellular pathways, involving induced proteins, other cytokines and target cells, are complex and have been only partially defined. Effects observed *in vitro* and in animal models have been poor predictors of patient responses, as they are often species specific. In dose–response studies, maximum activity is frequently not associated with the maximum tolerated dose, as expected from classical models. It is apparent that greater understanding of the cytokine network is required before cytokines achieve their full promise in clinical practice.

Interferon-α was the first recombinant protein to become available for cancer treatment. A wide variety of cytokines are now available for study, although relatively few have been approved for routine therapy

Table 10.1   Cytokines licensed for use in cancer therapy

Cytokine	Generic names	Licensed indications
Interferon-α	Interferon-α2a Interferon-α2b Interferon-αN1	Treatment of hairy cell leukaemia, CML, myeloma, follicular NHL, cutaneous cell lymphoma, AIDS-related Kaposi's sarcoma, metastatic renal cell carcinoma, metastatic melanoma, carcinoid syndrome
Interleukin 2	Aldesleukin	Treatment of renal cell carcinoma
G-CSF	Filgrastim Lenograstim	Reduction in depth and duration of chemotherapy-induced neutropenia, acceleration of myeloid recovery after bone marrow transplantation, mobilisation of blood progenitor cells for transplantation
GM-CSF	Molgramostim Sargramostim	Reduction in chemotherapy-induced neutropenia; acceleration of myeloid recovery after bone marrow transplantation
Erythropoietin	Epoietin-α Epoietin-β	Prevention and treatment of anaemia after platinum based chemotherapy

(Table 10.1). Here we outline the clinical applications of the interferons, interleukins and haemopoietic growth factors currently available.

Interferons

Interferons were discovered in 1957 and were originally recognised as antiviral agents. They were later found to have a wider range of properties, including growth regulation and immune modulation. Type I interferons (IFN-α and IFN-β) share about 45% homology at the nucleotide level, the genes for both being on the short arm of chromosome 9. They act through the same receptor and have strong antiviral effects as well as inhibiting growth in a wide range of target cells and inducing expression of high levels of MHC class I antigens on their cell surface. Interferon-γ is the only type II interferon and has no homology with type I. It is encoded on chromosome 12 and acts through a distinct receptor with different effects, including the induction of class II MHC antigens and macrophage activation (De Maeyer and de Maeyer-Guignard, 1994). Only interferon-α is currently licensed for cancer therapy.

The anti-cancer effects of interferon-α are mediated by direct antiproliferative effect on cells, altering oncogene expression and affecting differentiation pathways. It also acts indirectly on the immune system through activation of natural killer (NK) cells and macrophages, and by enhancing MHC expression on tumour cells, thus increasing their recognition by the immune system. The use of interferons in patients with chronic viral hepatitis can reduce the incidence of hepatocellular carcinoma (Nishiguchi *et al.*, 1995) and promises to be useful in preventing other virus-induced tumours.

Interferon-α became available for clinical use in 1981, and several preparations are now available (Table 10.1). IFN-α is administered daily or thrice weekly by subcutaneous (s.c.) injection in doses ranging from 1 to 36 MU/m^2. The most common adverse effect is a 'flu-like' syndrome, including fever, myalgia, headache and fatigue, which occurs up to 12 hours after injection and may be dose limiting but is often partially responsive to paracetamol. Other adverse effects are shown in Table 10.2.

Hairy cell leukaemia

IFN-α was licensed in 1986 for the treatment of this rare chronic B-cell leukaemia, which is characterised by splenomegaly, pancytopenia and opportunistic infections. Before this, splenectomy was the only effective treatment. The overall response rate for IFN-α is greater than 80%, with 40% complete response and a median duration of response of 24–30 months (Troussard and Flandrin, 1994). Although this has been the treatment of choice for the last decade, new cytotoxic agents such as the purine analogues pentostatin (2´-deoxycoformycin) and cladribine (2-chlorodeoxyadenosine) are now available and may supersede it (Gollard *et al.*, 1995; Mercieca *et al.*, 1996).

Chronic myeloid leukaemia

This leukaemia is characterised by the clonal expansion of myeloid cells bearing the 'Philadelphia' chromosome, a t(9;22) translocation, that apposes the proto-oncogene c-*abl* and the breakpoint cluster region *bcr*, producing a 201-kDa fusion protein with enhanced tyrosine kinase activity and the ability to transform cells (Yin *et al.*, 1995). Typically, the disease follows a chronic phase for several years before transformation to an accelerated phase that is rapidly fatal. Alkylating agents can

Table 10.2   Common adverse effects of interferon-α. The incidence of side-effects is dose and schedule dependent. It also depends on the underlying disease, e.g. myelosuppression is more common in patients with haematological malignancies

Side-effect	Incidence (%)
General	
Fever, chills	70–85
Malaise	75–100
Headache	50–90
Rash	20
Anorexia, weight loss	10–50
Alopecia	<5
Autoimmune thyroiditis	5–50
Cardiovascular	
Hypotension	<5
Gastrointestinal	
Nausea and vomiting	30–60
Diarrhoea	60
Neurological	
Fits	<5
Ataxia	<5
Encephalopathy	<5
Cortical blindness	Rare
Hepatotoxicity	
Increased serum transaminases	25–30
Hepatic necrosis	<5
Renal	
Proteinuria	5–20
Haematological	
Myelosuppression (anaemia, leucopenia, thrombocytopenia)	5–50

suppress the chronic phase, and myeloablative therapy with allogeneic bone marrow transplantation can sometimes eradicate the abnormal cell clone in selected patients. IFN-α can control the disease in about 70% and eliminate the t(9;22) clone in 10–20% of patients (Cirelli and Tyring, 1995). A recent Medical Research Council (MRC) study investigated the role of IFN-α in the chronic phase of the disease. Following induction chemotherapy, 587 patients were randomised to receive maintenance chemotherapy or IFN-α (3–12 MU/day). Median survival was significantly prolonged in patients receiving IFN-α (61 months versus 41 months) and 5-year survival was more likely in patients with a complete cytogenetic response (Allan *et al.*, 1995). Similar results were achieved in an Italian Co-operative Study (1994). Although IFN-α is now established in the therapy of the chronic phase of the disease, it is only moderately cost-effective (Liberato *et al.*, 1997). Whether further improvements in survival can be gained by combining cytotoxic treatments with interferons remains the subject of investigation.

Multiple myeloma

The conventional treatment of myeloma with alkylating agents and steroids with or without an anthracycline results in a response rate of about 50% and median survival of about 30 months. The response rate for single-agent IFN-α is poorer than with conventional chemotherapy. Induction therapy using a combination of cytotoxics and interferon has given mixed results, with some studies showing less disease progression and improved progression-free survival but others showing no difference (Cirelli and Tyring, 1995; Abrahamson *et al.*, 1996; Joshua *et al.*, 1997). In contrast, there are now persuasive data showing that maintenance treatment with IFN-α (2–5 MU, 3–5 times weekly) after remission induction with chemotherapy leads to significant extension of remission and, in some studies, superior overall survival (Mandelli *et al.*, 1990; Browman *et al.*, 1995; Westin *et al.*, 1995). This advantage can also be obtained in patients receiving maintenance interferon following high-dose therapy and haemopoietic stem cell transplantation (Cunningham *et al.*, 1993).

Lymphomas

Hodgkin's disease and high-grade non-Hodgkin's lymphomas can often be cured by conventional chemo-radiotherapy and the interferons are not used in their routine management. In contrast, low-grade non-Hodgkin's lymphoma is a chronic relapsing disease with a median survival of 6–10 years. It is sensitive to a variety of treatments, including radiation, single-agent alkylating agents, combination chemotherapy and interferons. The overall response rate to IFN-α alone is 40–50%, which is similar to the rates obtained with single-agent chemotherapy, but the responses are no more durable and the treatment is less well tolerated (Cirelli and Tyring, 1995). Several randomised studies have examined the role of IFN-α in combination with chemotherapy. Ozer *et al.* (1994) found that the added toxicity outweighed any benefit over chemotherapy alone, whereas other groups have achieved longer disease-free survival despite significant side-effects (Solal-Celigny *et al.*, 1993). Hagenbeek *et al.* (1995) assessed the use of IFN-α as maintenance therapy after induction chemotherapy and showed a significantly better progression-free survival in the IFN-α arm

(135 weeks versus 86 weeks). Early reports of the use of IFN-α as maintenance therapy after bone marrow transplantation, either alone or in combination with cyclosporin or IL-2, are encouraging (Gryn *et al.*, 1997; Nagler *et al.*, 1997).

Kaposi's sarcoma

Until the advent of AIDS, Kaposi's sarcoma was an unusual form of skin cancer that rarely involved the viscera. High doses of IFN-α (20–50 MU/m^2) were initially used in AIDS-related disease with a response rate of about 30% but high toxicity (Evans *et al.*, 1991). Subsequent studies have investigated low-dose IFN-α (2–3 MU/m^2) in combination with AZT and have shown response rates of between 40% and 60% with few side-effects (Mauss and Jablonowski, 1995; Fischl *et al.*, 1996).

Melanoma

The incidence of malignant melanoma has increased dramatically over the last few decades. It is relatively chemo- and radiotherapy insensitive, but rare spontaneous regressions suggest that immunological anti-tumour responses occasionally occur. In patients with metastatic disease, IFN-α alone gives response rates of 15–20%, similar to single-agent chemotherapy (Cirelli and Tyring, 1995). Most studies of IFN-α in combination with chemotherapy have shown no improvement in response rate, with increased toxicity (Schultz *et al.*,1997; Tamm *et al.*, 1997). The role of IFN-α in combination with IL-2 is being evaluated, and this is discussed below.

The immunomodulatory effect of IFN-α is likely to be greatest when there is minimal residual disease, and this is the rationale for using IFN-α as adjuvant therapy. Kirkwood *et al.* (1996) randomised 286 patients at high risk of relapse (i.e. with stage IIB and III disease) after curative surgery to observation or treatment with the maximum tolerated dose of IFN-α (20 MU/m^2/day i.v. for a month, followed by 10 MU/m^2 thrice weekly). Disease-free and overall survival were significantly increased in the IFN arm, but 67% of patients developed grade III toxicity. Patients at intermediate risk of relapse (stage IIA) have been shown to benefit from IFN-α therapy at doses as low as 3MU s.c. thrice weekly. Results from French and Austrian studies have shown improved disease free survival with greatly reduced toxicity. However, impact on overall survival remains unclear (Grob *et al.*, 1998; Pehamberger *et al.*, 1998).

Solid tumours

In metastatic renal cell carcinoma, the overall response rate to IFN-α alone is about 15%, with best results in patients with prior nephrectomy and of good performance status (Cirelli and Tyring, 1995). However, the combination of IFN-α and IL-2 appears more encouraging and is discussed below.

Initial clinical studies of IFN-α in colorectal cancer were promising, appearing to confirm *in vitro* demonstrations of synergy with 5-fluorouracil (5-FU). However, several large randomised studies comparing 5-FU and folinic acid with 5-FU and IFN-α showed no benefit in response rates or survival times with increased toxicity in the IFN-α arm (Corfu-A Study Group, 1995; Hill *et al.*, 1995).

Small cell lung cancer is initially chemosensitive but usually relapses. IFN-α is attractive as a maintenance therapy in patients with minimal residual disease. Although several Finnish studies have found significant survival benefit in patients treated with low-dose lymphoblastoid IFN-α as maintenance therapy (Mattson *et al.*, 1997), an American study failed to show a benefit in survival or time to progression in the IFN-α arm, largely because of the high discontinuation rate (43 of 64 patients), which was attributed to unacceptable toxicity (Kelly *et al.*, 1995).

Tumour necrosis factor

Tumour necrosis factor α (TNFα) is a 17-kDa protein produced predominantly by macrophages in response to infection and other cytokines. It has a myriad of biological effects, many of which are highly toxic to cells. It is also known as cachectin because of its ability to induce catabolism. TNF-α has been used as a single agent in phase I and II studies in cancer patients with disappointing results and high toxicity (Hieber and Heim, 1994).

Isolated limb perfusion, initially using single-agent melphalan, was first described 35 years ago as a treatment for melanomas and sarcomas limited to one limb. In the 1960s hyperthermia was added and was found to augment the response (Hafström and Mattsson, 1993). The addition of TNF-α and IFN-γ to melphalan in the perfusate appears to increase the response rate further to around 80% (Lienard *et al.*, 1994; Fraker *et al.*, 1996). Local toxicity includes skin, muscle and nerve damage with increased risk of vascular events. Thom *et al.* (1995) evaluated the toxicity using this technique administering IFN-γ, TNF and melphalan. They found that systemic leaks occurred in 6 of 19 patients and that all these patients developed hypotension requiring vasopressor support.

The interleukins

In contrast to most other agents used in cancer therapy, the interleukins do not have direct anti-tumour effects. They act indirectly through immune and haemopoietic effector cells. The principal characteristics and functions of the interleukins are shown in Table 10.3. Because of the complex interactions between them, their effects are context dependent. As a result, their clinical benefits and toxicities have proved unpredictable.

Interleukin 1

IL-1 exists in two forms, IL-1α and IL-1β, encoded on chromosome 2. The IL-1 receptor binds both forms and is encoded on the same chromosome. This cytokine has a broad spectrum of activity as a result of its ability to induce the expression of other cytokines and colony-stimulating factors. Much of the reported work is in animal models so the relevance to humans can only be extrapolated. However, IL-1 does appear to have several potential roles. Firstly, it has been shown to increase the number of colony-forming units of granulocyte–monocytes (CFU-GM) following bone marrow transplantation (Elkordy *et al.*, 1997) and carboplatin chemotherapy (Rinehart and Keville, 1997), so reducing the period of neutropenia. It has also been shown to enhance platelet recovery (Vadhan-Raj *et al.*, 1994a). Secondly, IL-1 has been shown to have direct anti-tumour activity in mice (Brunda *et al.*, 1994). Phase I studies administering IL-1 intravenously have been reported in patients with advanced cancer; dose-limiting toxicities were similar to those seen with IL-2 (Crown *et al.*, 1993). The anti-cancer of effect of IL-1 has been enhanced by the addition of IL-2, with increased lymphokine-activated killer (LAK) cell activity being shown in humans (Triozzi *et al.*, 1995).

Interleukin 2

IL-2 was first identified as a growth promoter for T cells. It is a 15.5-kDa glycoprotein encoded on chromosome 4 and is predominantly produced by activated T-helper cells. Binding of IL-2 to its specific receptor induces activation and proliferation of T cells, and also B lymphocytes, NK cells, monocytes and macrophages. In addition, the synthesis of other cytokines, particularly TNF and IFN-α, is enhanced (Goldsmith and Greene, 1994).

Table 10.3 Selected characteristics of the interleukins

Cytokine	Molecular weight	Principal sources	Target cells	Activities
IL-1α, IL-1β	18-kDa monomer	Monocytes, macrophages, B-cells, dendritic cells, endothelial cells, etc.	T_H cells	Co-stimulates activation, induces IL-2 production
			B cells	Promotes maturation and clonal expansion
			NK cells	Enhances activity
			Endothelial cells	Increases expression of ICAMs
			Macrophages and neutrophils	Chemotactically attracts
			Hepatocytes	Induces synthesis of acute-phase proteins
			Hypothalamus	Induces fever
IL-2	15-kDa monomer	T_H1 cells	Antigen-primed T_H and T_C cells	Induces proliferation
			Antigen-specific T-cell clones	Supports long-term growth
			NK (some) and T_C cells	Enhances activity
			B cells	Co-factor for growth and differentiation
IL-3	23-kDa monomer	T_H cells, NK cells, mast cells, keratinocytes, neuronal cells	Early haemopoietic cells	Supports growth and differentiation, synergises with stem cell factor
			Mast cells	Stimulates growth and histamine secretion
IL-4	18-kDa monomer	T_H2 cells, mast cells, bone marrow stroma	Antigen-primed B cell	Co-stimulates activation
			Activated B cells	Stimulates proliferation and activation, induces class switch to IgG1 and IgE
			Resting B cells	Up-regulates class II MHC expression
			Thymocytes and T cells	Induces proliferation
			Macrophages	Up-regulates class II MHC expression, increases phagocytic activity
			Mast cells	Stimulates growth
			Dendritic cells	Stimulates proliferation

(continue . . .)

Table 10.3 Continued

Cytokine	Molecular weight	Principal sources	Target cells	Activities
IL-5	50-kDa homodimer	T_H2 cells, mast cells	Activated B cell	Stimulates proliferation and differentiation, induces class switch to IgA
			Eosinophils	Promotes growth and differentiation
IL-6	26-kDa homodimer	Monocytes, macrophages, T_H2 cells, bone marrow stromal cells, fibroblasts, endothelial cells	Proliferating B cell	Promotes terminal differentiation into plasma cells
			Plasma cells	Stimulates antibody secretion
			Myeloid stem cells	Promotes differentiation of megakaryocytes
			Hepatocytes	Induces synthesis of acute-phase proteins
IL-7	25-kDa monomer	Bone marrow and thymic stromal cells, fetal liver	Lymphoid stem cells	Induces differentiation into progenitor B and T cells
			Resting T cells	Increases expression of IL-2 and its receptor
			B-cell precursors	Supports growth
			Monocytes	Induces cytokine secretion and tumoricidal activity
IL-8	6- to 15-kDa monomer/dimer	Monocytes, macrophages and endothelial cells	Neutrophils	Chemotactically attracts, induces adherence to vascular endothelium and extravasation into tissues
IL-9	40-kDa monomer	T_H cells	Some T_H cells	Mitogenic, supporting proliferation in absence of antigen
			B cells	Potentiates IL-4-induced IgE synthesis
			Erythroid precursors	Supports growth and differentiation

Interleukin	Structure	Source cells	Target cells	Functions
IL-10	32-kDa homodimer	T_H2 cells, B cells, macrophages	Macrophages Antigen-presenting cells	Suppresses cytokine production Down-regulates class II MHC expression
IL-11	23-kDa monomer	Bone marrow stromal cells	Plasmacytomas B-cell progenitor Megakaryocytes Hepatocytes	Supports growth Promotes differentiation Promotes proliferation and differentiation Induces synthesis of acute-phase proteins
IL-12	35- + 40-kD heterodimer	Macrophages, B cells	Activated TC cells NK and LAK cells and activated T_H1 cells	Acts synergistically with IL-2 to induce differentiation into cytotoxic T lymphocytes Stimulates proliferation
IL-13	14-kDa monomer	T_H cells	Macrophages B cells	Inhibits activation and release of inflammatory cytokines, important regulator of immune response Induces IgE synthesis
IL-14	468 amino acids	T cells	B cells	Induces proliferation, inhibits Ig secretion
IL-15	14 kDa		Binds to β-chain of IL-2 receptor	Stimulates T-cell proliferation and induction of LAK cells

The precise mechanism by which IL-2 exerts an anti-tumour response is not clearly defined, but it is likely to be indirect, by stimulation of cytotoxic T cells and NK cells and the production of other cytokines. In humans, the main tumour responses have been seen in melanoma and renal cell carcinomas (reviewed by Taneja *et al.*, 1995), both of which may also undergo spontaneous regression.

IL-2 can be given by subcutaneous or intravenous injection or infusion. Its toxicity has limited its widespread use in patients. The vast majority of patients are affected by the grade I/II toxicities commonly associated with other cytokines, including fever, nausea and vomiting, diarrhoea, fatigue, myalgia and arthralgia. Erythema at the site of injection is also common. The most severe toxicities occur at higher doses and are associated with a vascular leak syndrome, which is manifested by hypotension, tachycardia and oliguria, and can result in multiorgan damage (Table 10.4). This syndrome is thought to be mediated by nitric oxide produced in response to local secondary release of cytokines such as TNF, IL-1 and IFN-γ. A number of TNF inhibitors have been evaluated in order to reduce this but with little benefit (Margolin *et al.*, 1997). Autoimmune phenomena can occur following treatment with IL-2 (Gaspari, 1994). These include hypothyroidism, pemphigus, psoriasis and vitiligo. Haematological toxicities including defects in the coagulation pathways are common, and reversible renal dysfunction has also been reported.

IL-2 has been used as a single agent, but the optimal regimen remains uncertain. Metastatic renal cell carcinoma has a median survival of less than a year. IL-2 has been administered in this disease at high dose intravenously, as a bolus or continuous infusion, and at a low dose subcutaneously or intravenously (Taneja *et al.*, 1995). In 255 patients with metastatic renal cell carcinoma receiving high-dose intravenous therapy (6×10^5 IU/kg 8-hourly on days 1–5 and 15–19 every 6 weeks) the overall response rate was 14% with a median duration of response of 31 months. Toxicity was high, with 4% treatment-related deaths (Fyfe *et al.*, 1995, 1996). In metastatic melanoma, a response rate of 17% with duration of response of 7–91 months in the complete responders was obtained using IL-2 at 7.2×10^5 IU/kg (Rosenberg *et al.*, 1994).

High- and low-dose intravenous regimens were compared in a randomised study and gave similar response rates. However, toxicity was dramatically different, with hypotension requiring supportive care occurring in 52% of patients in the high-dose arm compared with only 3% of those receiving the lower doses (Yang *et al.*, 1994). Similar response rates and toxicity are obtained using continuous infusions

Table 10.4   Common adverse effects of IL-2 (after Fyfe *et al.*, 1995). The incidence of side-effects is dose and schedule dependent

Side-effect	Incidence (%)	
	Grade III/IV	All
General		
Fever	24	97
Oedema	2	55
Rash	1	25
Cardiovascular		
Hypotension	74	96
Arrhythmias	2	14
Myocardial ischaemia	2	2
Gastrointestinal		
Nausea and vomiting	25	89
Diarrhoea	22	81
Stomatitis	4	32
Gastrointestinal bleeding	3	15
Neurological		
Mental status change	28	82
Pulmonary		
Dyspnoea	17	57
Hepatic		
Abnormal liver function	9–21	70–85
Renal		
Oliguria	46	81
Raised creatinine	14	81
Haematological		
Thrombocytopenia	21	83
Anaemia	18	99

(Weiss *et al.*, 1992). Subcutaneous administration of low-dose IL-2 is associated with minimal toxicity and a reported response rate of 29% in one study of renal cell carcinoma (Lissoni *et al.*, 1994). It may, therefore, be possible to reduce toxicity dramatically with low-dose subcutaneous IL-2 therapy without sacrificing response rates. Several groups have looked for factors predictive of a good response to minimise the risk of therapy. In renal cell carcinoma, predictors of good response are a performance status of 0, previous nephrectomy, no prior immunotherapy, interval between diagnosis of the primary tumour and metastases of greater than a year and metastases outside the liver (Lissoni *et al.*, 1994; Fyfe *et al.*, 1995; Royal *et al.*, 1996). In melanoma, the only reported predictor of good response is the sole presence of subcutaneous metastases (Royal et al., 1996).

In 1985, Rosenberg et al. reported a response rate of 44% in patients with metastatic cancer using high-dose IL-2 and autologous LAK cells, most responses occurring in renal cell tumours and melanoma. This report paved the way for a large number of studies examining the role of IL-2 in these tumour types (Rosenberg, 1992). In mice, IL-2 showed anti-tumour activity both alone and with LAK cells, the greatest benefit of additional LAK cells being seen in combination with the lowest doses of IL-2. In patients, LAK cells are generated by administering IL-2 for several days prior to leukapheresis. The lymphocytes are isolated by Ficoll–Hypaque gradient centrifugation, cultured for 3–4 days with IL-2 and harvested before reinfusion. This process is time-consuming and carries a risk of infection. In 181 patients with advanced disease randomised to receive high-dose IL-2 with or without LAK cells, there was a trend towards improved survival in the IL-2/LAK cell arm in patients with melanoma, but no such trend in renal cell carcinoma (Rosenberg et al., 1993). Following this, the combined IL-2/LAK regimen lost favour.

Interest turned to the use of tumour-infiltrating lymphocytes (TILs) in combination with IL-2. TILs are generated ex vivo from tumour biopsies, which is time-consuming, expensive and not always feasible. It is possible to generate populations of almost pure CD8+ cells with highly specific anti-tumour cytolytic activity. The combination of TILs and IL-2 has been used in metastatic melanoma, ovarian tumours and non-small cell lung cancer (Rosenberg et al., 1988; Ratto et al., 1995). Using TILs and moderate-dose IL-2 produced response rates in metastatic melanoma comparable to high-dose IL-2 alone but without the associated toxicities (Goedegebuure et al., 1995). It is hoped that TILs transfected with DNA encoding IL-2 will prove both more effective and less toxic.

In an attempt to improve response rates, IL-2 and IFN-α have been studied in combination. It is postulated that IFN-α will up-regulate MHC class I expression and tumour-associated antigens on tumour cells, which may then be destroyed by the IL-2-activated lymphocytes. Animal studies suggested that such synergy did occur, and an initial study of high-dose IL-2 and IFN-α reported a response rate of 31% in patients with renal cell carcinoma (Rosenberg et al., 1989). The dose of each cytokine required to achieve responses in man remains unclear. Several groups have studied high-dose IL-2 in combination with IFN-α. A comparison of high-dose bolus IL-2 (24×10^6 IU/m^2) with IL-2 (14.4×10^6 IU/m^2) in combination with IFN-α (3×10^6 IU/m^2 8-hourly on days 1–5 and 15–19) in renal cell carcinoma showed that response rates (17% and 11% respectively) were not significantly different, but response duration was superior with IL-2 alone. The high toxicity of the two treatments was comparable (Atkins *et al.*, 1993). Marincola *et al.* (1995) reported on patients with melanoma, renal cell carcinoma and colorectal tumours treated with escalating doses of IL-2 and IFN-α. The overall response rate was 23%, and the 5-year survival rate was 25% for renal cell carcinoma and 6% for melanoma. It was concluded that the highest dose of IFN-α was associated with the highest response rate but that this did not result in improved survival and any potential benefit was outweighed by the increased toxicity.

Phase I and II studies of lower dose IL-2 as a continuous infusion in combination with IFN-α gave similar results to high-dose treatment (West *et al.*, 1990; Ilson *et al.*, 1992). European groups have favoured the use of low-dose subcutaneous IL-2 in combination with IFN-α, as it is better tolerated (Atzpodien *et al.*, 1991). In a phase II study using IL-2 1.5×10^6 IU/m^2/day for 5 days a week and IFN-α 1.5×10^6 IU/m^2/ day, response rates of up to 24% have been reported in patients with renal cell carcinoma with acceptable toxicity (Gause *et al.*, 1996). This regimen appears to offer a practicable alternative to single-agent high-dose IL-2 approved in the USA.

The combination of IL-2 with chemotherapy, so-called biochemotherapy, has been reported in patients with metastatic melanoma. Results to date indicate that the addition of IL-2 can increase the response rate, but no survival benefits have been demonstrated (Guida *et al.*, 1996; Legha *et al.*, 1996; Legha, 1997; Keilholz *et al.*, 1997). Further studies are needed to compare biochemotherapy and chemotherapy directly.

In summary, IL-2 has demonstrable activity in both melanoma and renal cell carcinoma, with response rates of 12–25%. Administration at low doses subcutaneously appears as effective as high-dose intravenous therapy and less toxic. The combination of IL-2 with IFN-α is well tolerated at lower doses, although whether the combination significantly improves response or survival is unproven. The use of IL-2 and chemotherapy requires further assessment.

In haematological malignancies there has been great interest in using IL-2 as an immunomodulator following high-dose therapy and bone marrow transplantation. It is recognised that patients who develop a graft-versus-host (GVH) response after receiving allogeneic bone marrow can also exhibit a graft-versus-leukaemia response that may eradicate minimal residual disease and improve survival. Administration of IL-2 immediately after allogeneic transplantation can reduce the incidence of GVH, whereas later administration can increase it and can actually induce it in autologous transplantation. Early studies have been encouraging, but this remains an experimental treatment (Higuchi *et al.*, 1991; Soiffer *et al.*, 1992; Hamon *et al.*, 1993).

A further area of research interest is that of transfecting tumour cells with the gene for IL-2. In experimental studies, a high level of IL-2 expression resulted in tumour regression, and this was found to be dependent on CD8⁺ T cells (Fearon *et al.*, 1990). However, in CD8-depleted mice there is evidence that tumour formation is delayed, suggesting that another cell type plays an important role, and it has been postulated that NK cells are involved. A phase I clinical study has recently been reported, using autologous tumour cells given with IL-2-transfected fibroblasts as a vaccine, and this has been shown to enhance specific anti-tumour cytotoxic T-cell responses (Veelken *et al.*, 1997). Co-administration of IL-2 with DNA vaccines has been evaluated as a means to increase the immunogenicity of DNA vaccines for infectious diseases and cancer therapy. In an experimental murine tumour model, administration of recombinant IL-2 greatly enhanced the effects of DNA immunisation (Irvine *et al.*, 1996; McLaughlin *et al.*, 1996). Other cytokines, such as GM-CSF and IL-12, have also been used as adjuvants to DNA vaccines (Conry *et al.*, 1996). These novel techniques have far from widespread use, but offer exciting opportunities to reduce the systemic toxicities seen with current cytokine therapy.

Interleukin 4

IL-4 exists in three variants, all encoded by the same gene on chromosome 5. It is predominantly secreted by T lymphocytes and mast cells. It has a wide range of actions on B cells, T cells and NK cells, as well as haemopoietic cells (Banchereau and Rybak, 1994). Studies in mice have shown a potent anti-tumour response (Tepper *et al.*, 1992). In human studies, an increase in peripheral eosinophil counts has been seen, although the relevance of this in terms of anti-tumour effect is uncertain (Sosman *et al.*, 1994). Phase I studies using recombinant IL-4 given intravenously and subcutaneously have reported a maximum tolerated dose of 10–15 μg/kg/day intravenously (Atkins *et al.*, 1992; Gilleece *et al.*, 1992). The toxicities included a 'flu-like syndrome, headache and abnormal liver function tests. However, the results of two phase II studies of IL-4 in 49 patients with metastatic melanoma or renal cell carcinoma showed no meaningful anti-tumour activity (Margolin *et al.*, 1994).

Interleukin 6

IL-6 is encoded on chromosome 7 and acts through a specific receptor. It has multiple biological effects, including the regulation of haemopoiesis, immune responses and acute-phase reactions. Numerous preclinical studies, *in vitro* and *in vivo*, indicate that IL-6 is a potent megakaryocyte maturation factor. Differentiation of both B and cytotoxic T cells is mediated by IL-6, as is production of IL-2 and its receptor (Hirano, 1994). Recent work with IL-6 'knockout' mice suggests that its predominant physiological role may be that of an immune regulator. Defects in the regulation of the acute-phase response and the lymphoid system were seen in these animals, but there was little effect on haemopoiesis (Kopf *et al.*, 1994). Because of its many indirect actions, there has been difficulty in predicting the clinical effects of IL-6 from preclinical data. Clinical studies are examining its role as a platelet growth factor and as an anti-tumour agent. In animal models, IL-6 increases platelet counts. Phase I studies have reported the safe use of this cytokine in patients, with accelerated platelet recovery following chemotherapy (D'Hondt *et al.*, 1995; Veldhuis *et al.*, 1995).

IL-6 is capable of stimulating the growth of a number of tumour cell lines, including myeloma, mesothelioma and ovarian tumours. Indeed, it functions as an autocrine growth factor in Castleman's disease. The use of anti-IL-6 antibodies has been described to reduce tumour bulk in a murine mesothelioma model (Bielefeldt *et al.*, 1995). Sosman *et al.* (1997) reported a phase I study in patients with solid tumours, with no objective responses seen. Side-effects such as chills, fever, fatigue, confusion and reversible changes in liver function have been reported. The dose-limiting toxicities appear to be neurological events, including confusion, blurred vision, ataxia and proximal weakness.

Interleukin 10

IL-10 is produced by monocytes and certain B cells, and acts on many cell types. It inhibits the synthesis of other cytokines and stimulates mast cell and B-cell growth, while suppressing T-cell growth. These properties suggest that IL-10 would have marked anti-inflammatory effects, and *in vivo* it has been shown to protect against endotoxaemia. It has also been proposed that the expression of IL-10 may influence tumour growth and metastatic capacity. Huang *et al.* (1996) injected mice with a human melanoma cell line transfected with the gene for IL-10. A marked reduction in tumour growth and metastases which correlated with reduced neovascularity was observed.

Haemopoietic growth factors

Haemopoiesis is regulated by a network of growth factors that act on bone marrow progenitors. Some, such as IL-3 and stem cell factor (SCF), act on primitive blood progenitor cells and stimulate proliferation of a wide range of haemopoietic cells. Others, such as erythropoietin and G-CSF, act on more mature, lineage-specific progenitors, promoting the growth and differentiation of particular cell types. Like the other cytokines, the haemopoietic growth factors were purified in minute amounts from biological materials in the 1970s, but became available for clinical use only after cloning and recombinant production in the late 1980s. Many are still undergoing clinical evaluation.

Erythropoietin

Erythropoietin is a 30-kDa glycoprotein, produced by peritubular cells in the kidney in response to hypoxia. It binds to specific receptors on primitive and committed erythroid progenitor cells in the bone marrow, stimulating erythrocyte production. Recombinant erythropoietin is widely used to treat anaemia in patients with chronic renal failure (Erslev, 1991). More recently, it has been licensed for use in the anaemia associated with platinum-containing chemotherapy. Erythropoietin is given by subcutaneous injection, conventionally thrice weekly, at doses of 50–300 IU/kg. It is associated with few adverse events, but pain at the injection site and facial flushing can occur. Increased blood pressure, polycythaemia and thrombocytosis can rarely cause thrombosis. Adequate iron stores are needed to obtain a response to erythropoietin.

Malignant disease is frequently accompanied by a normochromic normocytic anaemia, which may be exacerbated by chemotherapy. Such patients have inappropriately low serum erythropoietin. Cisplatin impairs erythropoietin production by causing progressive damage to the renal tubules, further blunting the response to anaemia. Early studies examined the effect of erythropoietin in patients receiving cisplatin who were already anaemic and found that their haematocrit rose significantly. In a placebo-controlled study in patients with cisplatin-associated anaemia, blood transfusion was required less often in patients receiving erythropoietin 100 U/kg s.c. thrice weekly (20% versus 56%) (Cascinu *et al.*, 1994). In non-platinum chemotherapy-induced anaemia, studies have also shown significant rises in haematocrit and reductions in transfusion requirements (Platanias *et al.*, 1991). Ludwig *et al.* (1995) found similar benefits in anaemic cancer patients who had not received chemotherapy. Most studies have determined response by laboratory parameters and transfusion requirements, whereas only a few studies have examined the effect of erythropoietin on quality of life. These demonstrate increased energy levels and well-being in the groups treated with erythropoietin (Case *et al.*, 1993; Leitgeb *et al.*, 1994).

Because erythropoietin use reduces the hazards of blood transfusion, it is attractive in countries without a secure supply of screened blood. The cost-effectiveness of treatment is difficult to assess: a study from the USA compared the cost of erythropoietin with blood transfusion; 64% of erythropoietin recipients responded at a cost of $12 971 per patient, whereas 100% of patients receiving blood responded at a cost of $4481 (Sheffield *et al.*, 1997). This study, however, compared only the healthcare costs and did not take into account broader economic considerations such as work days lost.

Thrombopoietin

Thrombopoietin (*c-mpl* ligand, megakaryocyte growth and development factor, MGDF) is a 70-kDa glycoprotein encoded on chromosome 3. It is produced by hepatocytes and bone marrow and is essential for the proliferation, differentiation and maturation of megakaryocytes into platelets (Kaushansky, 1995). In animal studies, administration of recombinant thrombopoietin leads to a dose-dependent increase in platelet and megakaryocyte numbers (Akahori *et al.*, 1996). The first clinical studies have now been reported. In a phase I study, a single dose of intravenous thrombopoietin gave a dose-related increase in platelets beginning at day 4 and peaking at day 12, accompanied by an increase in megakaryocytes and other bone marrow progenitors (Vadhan-Raj *et al.*, 1997). The platelets had normal morphology and function. No significant adverse effects were reported. In a larger placebo-controlled study, MGDF was given subcutaneously in multiple doses following chemotherapy. Platelet numbers were significantly higher in the MGDF arm. The majority of adverse events related to the concurrent chemotherapy, although one patient with thrombocytosis did develop a pulmonary embolism (Fanucchi *et al.*, 1997). These early findings suggest that thrombopoietin is likely to be useful in the prevention and treatment of chemotherapy-induced thrombocytopenia. Other potential roles may be in mobilisation of progenitor cells for blood progenitor cell transplantation, or in the apheresis of normal donors.

Interleukin 11

IL-11 is a recently identified haemopoeitic growth factor, acting mainly on megakaryocyte maturation and platelet production. In preclinical studies, enhanced platelet recovery was seen after intensive chemotherapy and bone marrow transplantation. A phase I trial in patients with breast cancer found the maximum tolerated dose to be 75 μg/kg. The dose-limiting toxicities included myalgia and fatigue; other adverse effects included weight gain and oedema. Patients receiving more than 25 μg/kg had fewer episodes of thrombocytopenia (Gordon *et al.*, 1996). Tepler *et al.* (1996) studied 93 patients who had previously required platelet transfusions and were randomised to receive placebo or IL-11 at a dose of either 25 or 50 μg/kg after chemotherapy. Of those treated with 50 μg/kg, 30% of patients did not require platelet transfusion compared with only 4% in the placebo arm. There were, however, no significant differences in neutrophil count and hospitalisation time between the two arms.

Myeloid colony-stimulating factors

Granulocyte–macrophage colony-stimulating factor (GM-CSF) is a 15- to 32-kDa glycoprotein encoded by a gene on chromosome 5, close to those for IL-3, IL-4, IL-5 and M-CSF. Chromosome deletions in this area are common in myelodysplasia and acute myelogenous leukaemia. GM-CSF is produced by endothelial cells, fibroblasts and activated macrophages. The receptors comprise a specific α-chain and a β-chain that is shared with the IL-3 receptor. GM-CSF acts on committed myeloid progenitors to stimulate the production of granulocytes, macrophages, eosinophils and basophils. It also acts in synergy with IL-3 to increase multipotential and megakaryocyte colony formation (Lieschke and Burgess, 1992). Interestingly, transgenic GM-CSF-deficient mice have normal blood and bone marrow but demonstrate abnormalities in surfactant clearance in the lungs (Dranoff *et al.*, 1994).

G-CSF is a 19-kDa glycoprotein encoded by a gene on chromosome 17. Like GM-CSF, it is produced by a variety of cells, but its receptors are more restricted in their distribution and G-CSF predominantly stimulates the proliferation, differentiation and activation of granulocytes (Lieschke and Burgess, 1992). As might be expected, transgenic G-CSF-deficient mice are granulocytopenic (Lieschke *et al.*, 1994).

Recombinant GM-CSF and G-CSF are available in glycosylated and non-glycosylated forms, but the clinical significance of these differences is unclear. They are typically administered subcutaneously. GM-CSF can cause fever, myalgia, bone pain and skin rashes. The most common side-effect of G-CSF is bone pain, which is usually mild and rarely requires discontinuation of treatment. These growth factors have two main roles in cancer therapy, to ameliorate myelotoxicity following chemotherapy and to mobilise blood progenitor cells for transplantation after high-dose therapy.

Both G-CSF and GM-CSF can reduce the depth and duration of neutropenia following conventional chemotherapy (Crawford *et al.*, 1991). This results in fewer episodes of neutropenic sepsis with some reduction in antibiotic use and inpatient days. Patients receiving growth factor support are more likely to receive their chemotherapy at full dose and on time. Attempts to support increased cytotoxic dose intensity have shown that modest increases are possible, and studies are in progress to determine whether this leads to better patient survival (Woll *et al.*, 1995).

The cost of prophylactic G-CSF or GM-CSF can rarely be justified with routine chemotherapy. Indeed, prophylactic antibiotics may be a cheaper and more effective alternative (Rodriguez *et al.*, 1990). The interventional use of myeloid growth factors in patients with established neutropenic sepsis can accelerate neutrophil recovery but does not lead to savings in antibiotic use or days in hospital (Biesma *et al.*, 1990; Maher *et al.*, 1994).

High-dose therapy with bone marrow or blood progenitor cell (BPC) transplantation is increasingly used in the treatment of leukaemias, lymphomas and selected solid tumours. G-CSF and GM-CSF can significantly shorten the period of profound neutropenia following transplantation, with consequent reductions in antibiotic use, although thrombocytopenia remains limiting (Gisselbrecht *et al.*, 1994). The finding that haemopoietic growth factors can mobilise BPC from the bone marrow into the peripheral blood has revolutionised high-dose therapy (Pettengell and Testa, 1995). Peripheral BPC can be collected by apheresis and used for transplantation. This has marked advantages over the use of bone marrow: apheresis is an outpatient procedure that does not require an anaesthetic, and the recovery of both neutrophils and platelets is accelerated following BPC transplantation, making the procedure shorter and safer (Schmitz *et al.*, 1996).

Interleukin 3

The gene for IL-3 is on chromosome 5 and encodes a 14- to 28-kDa glycoprotein that is produced by activated T cells, NK cells and mast cells. Preclinical studies have shown that IL-3 (multi-CSF) stimulates the growth and differentiation of multiple blood cell lineages and primitive pluripotent stem cells, often acting synergistically with other cytokines (Schrader, 1994). This raised hopes that it would ameliorate all the myelotoxic effects of anti-cancer treatments. Early clinical studies evaluated the safety, tolerability and activity of IL-3 following chemotherapy and demonstrated accelerated recovery of both neutrophil and platelet counts, with fewer treatment delays (D'Hondt *et al.*, 1993; Rinehart *et al.*, 1995). The maximum tolerated dose is 5 μg/kg/day given subcutaneously, with dose-limiting adverse effects including fever, fatigue and headaches (Rinehart *et al.*, 1995). It is less well tolerated than G-CSF or thrombopoietin.

Animal models have suggested that synergy between IL-3 and G-CSF/GM-CSF leads to optimal myelopoiesis. This led to the development of a novel recombinant fusion protein PIXY-321, which combines the active domains of GM-CSF and IL-3. The side-effects are those of its components. A phase I/II study showed that doses of 500–1000 μg/m^2/day prevented cumulative thrombocytopenia after two cycles of chemotherapy, and patients had higher nadir platelet counts than historical controls treated with GM-CSF alone (Vadhan-Raj *et al.*, 1994b). A randomised trial comparing PIXY-321 with GM-CSF in 53 patients showed no difference between the two arms in terms of nadir platelet counts, duration of thrombocytopenia or transfusion requirements, although the period of neutropenia was shorter in patients receiving PIXY-321 (O'Shaughnessy *et al.*, 1996). The sequential use of IL-3 and GM-CSF/G-CSF has been reported to improve platelet recovery in patients with prolonged chemotherapy-induced thrombocytopenia (Farber *et al.*, 1997).

IL-3 alone is a weak mobiliser of BPC. As predicted from animal models, it acts synergistically with late-acting haemopoietic growth factors to mobilise BPC, although it is unclear whether this offers any practical advantage over, for example, G-CSF alone (Pettengell and Testa, 1995; Ghielmini *et al.*, 1996).

Early-acting haemopoietic growth factors

Stem cell factor (SCF) is the ligand for the tyrosine kinase receptor encoded by the *c-kit* proto-oncogene, which is expressed on primitive and mature haemopoietic progenitor cells. SCF prevents apoptosis of progenitor cells and in combination with other cytokines facilitates their differentiation and maturation. SCF has limited efficacy when used alone but it acts synergistically with late-acting haemopoietic growth factors, such as G-CSF, to mobilise CD34+ progenitor cells (Weaver *et al.*, 1996; Moskowitz *et al.*, 1997). SCF has also been used in combination with IL-11 and G-CSF for *ex vivo* expansion of progenitor cells (Holyoake *et al.*, 1996; Cesana *et al.*, 1997). The use of SCF at high doses has been limited by the release of histamine from activated mast cells, but lower doses and premedication with antihistamines and β-agonists are better tolerated. Although these early studies show great promise, further evaluation both *in vitro* and *in vivo* is required before more widespread use.

Another early-acting haemopoietic growth factor that shows promise is FLK-2 (*flt-3* ligand). This stimulates the growth of marrow stem cells, T cells and dendritic cells. Unlike SCF, it does not cause mast-cell degranulation. Early clinical studies suggest that it will be better tolerated than stem cell factor.

Conclusions

This is by no means an exhaustive review but outlines the main roles for cytokines and growth factors that are currently licensed for clinical use. It has also touched on areas of current research in these and other more recently discovered cytokines. Although current clinical studies have not shown dramatic responses, the effects seen *in vitro* suggest that further understanding into the mechanism of action will enable future use to be enhanced. In particular, the use of cytokines in minimal residual disease, when the immune system is likely to be most capable of destroying remaining tumour cells, seems to be one of the ways to improve responses.

References

Abrahamson G M, Bird J M, Newland A C, *et al.* (1996) A randomized study of VAD therapy with either concurrent or maintenance interferon in patients with newly diagnosed multiple myeloma. *Br J Haematol* 94: 659–664.

Akahori H, Shibuya K, Obuchi M, *et al.* (1996) Effect of recombinant human thrombopoietin in non-human primates with chemotherapy-induced thrombocytopenia. *Br J Haematol* 94: 722–728.

Allan N C, Richards S M, Shepherd P C A, *et al.* (1995) UK Medical Research Council randomised, multicentre trial of interferon-alpha for chronic myeloid leukaemia: improved survival irrespective of cytogenetic response. *Lancet* 345: 1392–1397.

Atkins M B, Vachino G, Tilag H J, *et al.* (1992) Phase I evaluation of thrice daily intravenous bolus interleukin-4 in patients with refractory malignancy. *J Clin Oncol* 10: 1802–1809.

Atkins M B, Sparano J, Fisher R I, *et al.* (1993) Randomized phase II trial of high-dose interleukin-2 either alone or in combination with interferon alfa-2b in advanced renal cell carcinoma. *J Clin Oncol* 11: 661–670.

Atzpodien J, Poliwoda H, Kirchner H (1991) Alpha-interferon and interleukin-2 in renal cell carcinoma: Studies in non-hospitalised patients. *Semin Oncol* 18: 108–112.

Banchereau J, Rybak M E (1994) Interleukin-4. In: Thomson A, ed. *The Cytokine Handbook*, 2nd edn. London: Academic Press, 99–126.

Bielefeldt, Ohmann H, Marzo A L, *et al.* (1995) Interleukin-6 involvement in mesothelioma pathobiology: inhibition by interferon alpha immunotherapy. *Cancer Immunol Immunopathol* 40: 241–250.

Biesma B, De Vries E G E, Willemse P H B, *et al.* (1990) Efficacy and tolerability of recombinant human GM-CSF in patients with chemotherapy-related leukopenia and fever. *Eur J Cancer* 26: 932–936.

Browman G P, Bergsagel D, Sicheri D, *et al.* (1995) Randomized trial of interferon maintenance in multiple myeloma: a study of the National Cancer Institute of Canada clinical trials group. *J Clin Oncol* 13: 2354–2360.

Brunda M J, Wright R B, Luistro L, *et al.* (1994) Enhanced anti-tumor efficacy in mice by combination treatment with interleukin-1 and interferon alpha. *J Immunol* 152: 2324–2332.

Cascinu S, Fedeli A, Del Ferro E, *et al.* (1994) Recombinant human erythropoietin treatment in cisplatin-associated anaemia: a randomized, double-blind trial with placebo. *J Clin Oncol* 12: 1058–1062.

Case D C, Bukowski R M, Carey R W, *et al.* (1993) Recombinant human erythropoietin therapy for anaemic patients on combination chemotherapy. *J Natl Cancer Inst* 85: 801–806.

Cesana C, Carlostella C, Mangoni L, *et al.* (1997) In vitro growth of mobilised peripheral blood progenitor cells is significantly enhanced by stem cell factor. *Stem Cells* 15: 207–213.

Cirelli R, Tyring S K (1995) Major therapeutic uses of interferons. *Clin Immunother* 3: 27–87.

Conry R M, Widera G, LoBuglio A F, *et al.* (1996) Selected strategies to augment polynucleotide immunization. *Gene Therapy* 3: 67–74.

Corfu-A Study Group (1995) Phase III randomized study of two fluorouracil combinations with either interferon alfa-2a or leucovorin for advanced colorectal cancer. *J Clin Oncol* 13: 921–928.

Crawford J, Ozer H, Stroller R, *et al.* (1991) Reduction by G-CSF of fever and neutropenia induced by chemotherapy in patients with SCLC. *N Engl J Med* 315: 164–170.

Crown J, Jakubowski A, Gabrilove J (1993) Interleukin-1: biological effects in human haematopoiesis. *Leuk Lymphoma* 9: 433–440.

Cunningham D, Powles R, Malpas J S, *et al.* (1993) A randomized trial of maintenance therapy with intron A following high dose melphalan and ABMT in myeloma. *Proc Am Soc Clin Oncol* 12: 364.

De Maeyer E, De Maeyer-Guignard J (1994) Interferons. In: Thomson A, ed. *The Cytokine Handbook*, 2nd edn. London: Academic Press, 265–288.

D'Hondt V, Weynants P, Humblet Y, *et al.* (1993) Dose-dependent interleukin-3 stimulation of thrombopoiesis and neutropoiesis in patients with small-cell lung carcinoma before and following chemotherapy: a placebo controlled randomised phase 1b study. *J Clin Oncol* 11: 2063–2071.

D'Hondt V, Humblet Y, Guillaume T, *et al.* (1995) Thrombopoietic effects and toxicity of interleukin-6 in patients with ovarian cancer before and after chemotherapy: a multicentre placebo-controlled, randomized phase Ib trial. *Blood* 85: 2347–2353.

Dranoff G, Crawford A D, Sadelain M, *et al.* (1994) Involvement of granulocyte–macrophage colony-stimulating factor in pulmonary homeostasis. *Science* 264: 713–716.

Elkordy M, Crump M, Vredenburgh J J, *et al.* (1997) A phase I trial of recombinant human interleukin-1 beta following high-dose chemotherapy and autologous bone marrow transplantation. *Bone Marrow Transplant* 19: 315–322.

Erslev A J (1991) Erythropoietin. *N Engl J Med* 324: 1339–1344.

Evans L M, Itri L M, Campion M, *et al.* (1991) Interferon-α2a in the treatment of acquired immunodeficiency syndrome-related Kaposi's sarcoma. *J Immunother* 10: 39–50.

Fanucchi M, Glaspy J, Crawford J, *et al.* (1997) Effects of polyethylene glycol-conjugated recombinant human megakaryocyte growth and development factor on platelet counts after chemotherapy for lung cancer. *N Engl J Med* 336: 404–409.

Farber L, Haus U, Fuchsel G, *et al.* (1997) Treatment of prolonged chemotherapy induced severe thrombocytopenia with recombinant human interleukin-3: a report on four cases. *Anti-Cancer Drugs* 8: 288–292.

Fearon E, Pardoll D, Itaya T, *et al.* (1990) Interleukin-2 production by tumor cells bypasses T helper function in the generation of an anti-tumor response. *Cell* 60: 397–403.

Fischl M A, Finkelstein D M, He W (1996) A phase II study of recombinant human IFNα-2a and zidovidine in patients with AIDS related Kaposi's sarcoma. *J AIDS Human Retrovirol* 11: 379–384.

Fraker D L, Alexander H R, Andrich M, *et al.* (1996) Treatment of patients with melanoma of the extremity using hyperthermic isolated limb perfusion with melphalan, tumor necrosis factor, and interferon γ: results of a tumor necrosis factor dose-escalation study. *J Clin Oncol* 14: 479–489.

Fyfe G, Fisher R I, Rosenberg S A, *et al.* (1995) Results of treatment of 255 patients with metastatic renal cell carcinoma who received high-dose recombinant interleukin-2 therapy. *J Clin Oncol* 13: 688–696.

Fyfe G, Fisher R I, Rosenberg S A, *et al.* (1996) Long-term response data of 255 patients with metastatic renal cell carcinoma treated with high-dose recombinant interleukin-2 therapy. *J Clin Oncol* 14: 2410–2411.

Gaspari A A (1994) Autoimmunity as a complication of interleukin-2 immunotherapy. *Arch Dermatol* 30: 894–898.

Gause B L, Sznol M, Kopp W C, *et al.* (1996) Phase I study of subcutaneously administered interleukin-2 in combination with interferon alfa-2a in patients with advanced cancer. *J Clin Oncol* 14: 2234–2241.

Ghielmini M, Pettengell R, Coutinho L H, *et al.* (1996) The effect of the GM-CSF/IL-3 fusion protein PIXY321 on bone marrow and circulating haemopoietic cells of previously untreated patients with cancer. *Br J Haematol* 93: 6–12.

Gilleece M H, Scarffe J H, Ghosh A, *et al.* (1992) Recombinant interleukin-4 given as daily subcutaneous injections – a phase I dose toxicity trial. *Br J Cancer* 66: 204–210.

Gisselbrecht C, Prentice H G, Bacigalupo A, *et al.* (1994) Placebo-controlled phase III trial of lenograstim in bone marrow transplantation. *Lancet* 343: 696–700.

Goedegebuure P S, Douville L M, Li H, *et al.* (1995) Adoptive immunotherapy with tumor-infiltrating lymphocytes and interleukin-2 in patients with metastatic malignant melanoma and renal cell carcinoma. *J Clin Oncol* 13: 1939–1949.

Goldsmith M A, Greene W C (1994) Interleukin-2 and the interleukin-2 receptor. In: Thomson A, ed. *The Cytokine Handbook*, 2nd edn. London: Academic Press, 57–80.

Gollard R, Lee T C, Piro L D, *et al.* (1995) The optimal management of hairy cell leukaemia. *Drugs* 49: 921–931.

Gordon M S, McCaskill-Stevens W J, Battiato L A, *et al.* (1996) A phase I trial of recombinant interleukin-11 in women with breast cancer receiving chemotherapy. *Blood* 87: 3615–3624.

Grob J J, Dreno B, de la Salmoniere P, *et al.* (1998) Randomised trial of interferon α-2a as adjuvant therapy in resected primary melanoma thicker than 1.5 mm without clinically detectable node metastases. *Lancet* 351: 1905–1910.

Gryn J, Johnson E, Goldman N, *et al.* (1997) The treatment of relapsed or refractory intermediate grade non-Hodgkin's lymphoma with autologous bone marrow transplantation followed by cyclosporine and interferon. *Bone Marrow Transplant* 19: 221–226.

Guida M, Latorre A, Mastria A, *et al.* (1996) Subcutaneous recombinant interleukin-2 plus chemotherapy with cisplatin and dacarbazine in metastatic melanoma. *Eur J Cancer* 32A: 730–733.

Hafström L, Mattsson J (1993) Regional chemotherapy for malignant melanoma. *Cancer Treat Rev* 19: 17–28.

Hagenbeek A, Carde P, Somer R, *et al.* (1995) Interferon alfa-2a vs. control as maintenance therapy for low grade non-Hodgkin's lymphoma: results from a prospective randomized clinical trial. *Proc Am Soc Clin Oncol* 14: 386.

Hamon M D, Prentice H G, Gottlieb D J, *et al.* (1993) Immunotherapy with IL-2 after autologous bone marrow transplantation in AML. *Bone Marrow Transplant* 11: 199–401.

Hieber U, Heim M E (1994) Tumor necrosis factor for the treatment of malignancies. *Oncology* 51: 142–153.

Higuchi C M, Thompson J A, Peterson F B, *et al.* (1991) Toxicity and immuno-modulatory effects of IL-2 after autologous bone marrow transplantation for haematological malignancies. *Blood* 77: 2561–2268.

Hill M, Norman A, Cunningham D, *et al.* (1995) Royal Marsden phase III trial of fluorouracil with or without interferon alfa-2a in advanced colorectal cancer. *J Clin Oncol* 13: 1287–1302.

Hirano T (1994) Interleukin-6. In: Thomson A, ed. *The Cytokine Handbook*, 2nd edn. London: Academic Press, 145–168.

Holyoake T L, Freshney M G, McNair L, *et al.* (1996) *Ex vivo* expansion with stem cell factor and interleukin-11 augments both short term recovery post-trans-plant and the ability to serially transplant marrow. *Blood* 87: 4589–4595.

Huang S, Xie K, Bucana C D, *et al.* (1996) Interleukin-10 suppresses tumor growth and metastasis of human melanoma cells: potential inhibition of angiogene-sis. *Clin Cancer Res* 2: 1969–1979.

Ilson D H, Motzer R J, Kradin R L, *et al.* (1992) A phase II trial of interleukin-2 and interferon alfa-2a in patients with advanced renal cell carcinoma. *J Clin Oncol* 10: 1124–1130.

Irvine K R, Rao J B, Rosenberg S A, *et al.* (1996) Cytokine enhancement of DNA immunization leads to effective treatment of established pulmonary metas-tases. *J Immunol* 156: 238–245.

Italian Co-operative Study Group on Chronic Myeloid Leukaemia (1994) Interferon alfa-2a compared with conventional chemotherapy for the treatment of chronic myeloid leukaemia. *N Engl J Med* 330: 820–825.

Joshua D E, Penny R, Matthews J P, *et al.* (1997) Australian Leukaemia Study Group Myeloma II: a randomized trial of intensive combination chemotherapy with or without interferon in patients with myeloma. *Br J Haematol* 97: 38–45.

Kaushansky K (1995) Thrombopoietin: The primary regulator of platelet produc-tion. *Blood* 86: 419–431.

Keilholz U, Goey S H, Punt C J A, *et al.* (1997) Interferon alfa-2a and interleukin-2 with or without cisplatin in metastatic melanoma: a randomized trial of the European Organization for Research and Treatment of Cancer Melanoma Co-operative Group. *J Clin Oncol* 15: 2579–2588.

Kelly K, Crowley J J, Bunn P A, *et al.* (1995) Role of recombinant interferon alfa-2a maintenance in patients with limited-stage small-cell lung cancer respond-ing to concurrent chemoradiation: a Southwest Oncology Group study. *J Clin Oncol* 13: 2924–2930.

Kirkwood J M, Strawderman M H, Ernstoff M S, *et al.* (1996) Interferon alfa-2b adjuvant therapy of high-risk resected cutaneous melanoma: the Eastern Co-operative Oncology Group trial EST 1684. *J Clin Oncol* 14: 7–17.

Kopf M, Baumann H, Freer G, *et al.* (1994) Impaired immune and acute-phase responses in interleukin-6 deficient mice. *Nature* 368: 339–342.

Legha S S (1997) Durable complete responses in metastatic melanoma treated with interleukin-2 in combination with interferon-alfa and chemotherapy. *Semin Oncol* 24 (Suppl. 4): 39–43.

Legha S S, Ring S, Bedikian A, *et al.* (1996) Treatment of metastatic melanoma with combined chemotherapy containing cisplatin, vinblastine and dacarbazine (CVD) and biotherapy using interleukin-2 and interferon-α. *Ann Oncol* 7: 827–835.

Leitgeb C, Pechertorfer M, Fritz E, *et al.* (1994) Quality of life in chronic anaemia of cancer during treatment with recombinant human erythropoietin. *Cancer* 73: 2535–2542.

Liberato N L, Qaglini S, Barosi G (1997) Cost-effectiveness of interferon alfa in chronic myelogenous leukaemia. *J Clin Oncol* 15: 2673–2682.

Lienard D, Eggermont A M M, Schraffordt K (1994) Isolated perfusion of the limb with high dose tumor necrosis factor α, interferon γ and melphalan for melanoma stage III. Results of a multicentre study. *Melanoma Res* 4: 21–26.

Lieschke G J, Burgess A W (1992) Granulocyte colony-stimulating factor and granulocyte-macrophage colony-stimulating factor. *N Engl J Med* 327: 28–35, 99–106.

Lieschke G J, Grail D, Hodgson G, *et al.* (1994) Mice lacking in granulocyte colony-stimulating factor have chronic neutropenia, granulocyte and macrophage progenitor cell deficiency and impaired neutrophil mobilisation. *Blood* 84: 1737–1746.

Lissoni P, Barni S, Ardizzoia A, *et al.* (1994) Prognostic factors of the clinical response to subcutaneous immunotherapy with interleukin-2 alone in patients with metastatic renal cell carcinoma. *Oncology* 51: 59–62.

Ludwig H, Sundal E, Pechertorfer M, *et al.* (1995) Recombinant human erythropoietin for the correction of cancer associated anaemia with and without concomitant cytotoxic chemotherapy. *Cancer* 76: 2319–2329.

Maher D W, Lieschke G J, Green M, *et al.* (1994) Filgrastim in patients with chemotherapy-induced febrile neutropenia. A double-blind, placebo-controlled trial. *Ann Int Med* 121: 492–501.

Mandelli F, Avvisati G, Amadori S, *et al.* (1990) Maintenance treatment with recombinant interferon alfa-2b in patients with multiple myeloma responding to conventional induction chemotherapy. *N Engl J Med* 332: 1430–1434.

Margolin K, Aronson F R, Sznol M, *et al.* (1994) Phase II studies of recombinant human interleukin-4 in advanced renal cancer and malignant melanoma. *J Immunother* 15: 147–153.

Margolin K, Atkins M, Sparano J, *et al.* (1997) Prospective randomized trial of lisofylline for the prevention of toxicities of high-dose interleukin-2 therapy in advanced renal cancer and malignant melanoma. *Clin Cancer Res* 3: 565–572.

Marincola F M, White D E, Wise A P, *et al.* (1995) Combination therapy with interferon alfa-2a and interleukin-2 for the treatment of metastatic cancer. *J Clin Oncol* 13: 1110–1122.

Mattson K, Niiranen A, Ruotsalainen Y, *et al.* (1997) Interferon maintenance therapy for small cell lung cancer: Improvement in long term survival. *J Interferon Cytokine Res* 17: 103–105.

Mauss S, Jablonowski H (1995) Efficacy, safety and tolerance of low dose, long term interferon α and zidovidine in early stage AIDS associated Kaposi's sarcoma. *J AIDS Human Retrovirol* 10: 157–162.

McLaughlin J P, Schlom J, Kantor J A, *et al.* (1996) Improved immunotherapy of recombinant carcinoembryonic antigen vaccinia vaccine when given in combination with interleukin-2. *Cancer Res* 56: 2361–2367.

Mercieca J, Matutes E, Emmett E, *et al.* (1996) 2-Chlordeoxyadenosine in the treatment of hairy cell leukaemia: differences in the response in patients with and without abdominal lymphadenopathy. *Br J Haematol* 93: 409–411.

Moskowitz C H, Stiff P, Gordon M S, *et al.* (1997) Recombinant methionyl human stem cell factor and filgrastim for peripheral blood progenitor cell mobilisation and transplantation in non-Hodgkin's lymphoma patients – results of a phase I/II trial. *Blood* 89: 3136–3147.

Nagler A, Ackerstein A, Or R, *et al.* (1997) Immunotherapy with recombinant human interleukin-2 and recombinant interferon alfa in lymphoma patients post-autologous marrow or stem cell transplant. *Blood* 89: 3951–3959.

Nishigushi S, Kuroki T, Nakatani S, *et al.* (1995) Randomized trial of effects of interferon-α on incidence of hepatocellular carcinoma in chronic active hepatitis C with cirrhosis. *Lancet* 346: 1051–1055.

O'Shaughnessy J A, Tolcher A, Riseberg D, *et al.* (1996) Prospective, randomized trial of 5-fluorouacil, leucovorin, doxorubicin and cyclophosphamide chemotherapy in combination with interleukin-3/granulocyte-macrophage colony-stimulating factor (GM-CSF) fusion protein (PIXY321) versus GM-CSF in patients with advanced breast cancer. *Blood* 87: 2205–2211.

Ozer H, Anderson J H, Peterson B A, *et al.* (1994) Combination trial of recombinant human alpha-2a interferon and cyclophosphamide in follicular low grade non-Hodgkin's lymphoma. *Med Pediatr Oncol* 22: 228–235.

Pehamberger H, Soyer H P, Steiner A, *et al.* (1998) Adjuvant interferon alfa-2a treatment in resected primary stage II melanoma. *J Clin Oncol* 16: 1425–1429.

Pettengell R, Testa N G (1995) Biology of blood progenitor cells used in transplantation. *Int J Haematol* 61: 1–15.

Platanias L C, Miller C, Mick R, *et al.* (1991) Treatment of chemotherapy-induced anaemia with recombinant human erythropoietin in cancer patients. *J Clin Oncol* 9: 2021–2026.

Ratto G B, Melioli G, Zino P, *et al.* (1995) Immunotherapy with the use of tumor-infiltrating lymphocytes and interleukin-2 as adjuvant treatment in stage III non-small cell lung cancer. *J Thorac Cardiovasc Surg* 109: 1212–1217.

Rinehart J, Keville L R (1997) Reduction in carboplatin haemopoietic toxicity in tumor bearing mice: Comparative mechanisms and effects of interleukin-1b and corticosteroids. *Cancer Biotherapy Radiopharmaceuticals* 12: 101–109.

Rinehart J, Margolin K A, Triozzi P, *et al.* (1995) Phase I trial of recombinant interleukin-3 before and after carboplatin/etoposide chemotherapy in patients with solid tumors: a Southwest Oncology Group Study. *Clin Cancer Res* 1: 1139–1144.

Rodriguez M, Swan F, Hagemeister F, *et al.* (1990) High dose ESHAP with GM-CSF vs. prophylactic antibiotics. *Blood* 76 (Suppl. 1): 370a.

Rosenberg S A (1992) The immunotherapy and gene therapy of cancer. *J Clin Oncol* 10: 180–199.

Rosenberg S A, Lotze M T, Muul L M, *et al.* (1985) Observations on the systemic administration of autologous lymphokine-activated killer cells and recombinant interleukin-2 to patients with metastatic cancer. *N Engl J Med* 313: 1485–1492.

Rosenberg S A, Packard B S, Aebersold P M, *et al.* (1988) Use of tumor infiltrating lymphocytes and interleukin-2 in the immunotherapy of patients with metastatic melanoma: a preliminary report. *N Engl J Med* 319: 1676–1680.

Rosenberg S A, Lotze M T, Yang J C, *et al.* (1989) Combination therapy with interleukin-2 and alpha-interferon for the treatment of patients with advanced cancer. *J Clin Oncol* 7: 1863–1874.

Rosenberg S A, Lotze M T, Yang J C, et al. (1993) Prospective randomized trial of high-dose interleukin-2 alone or in conjunction with lymphokine-activated killer cells for the treatment of patients with advanced cancer. *J Natl Cancer Inst* 85: 622–632.

Rosenberg S A, Yang J C, Topialin S L, et al. (1994) Treatment of 283 consecutive patients with metastatic melanoma or renal cell cancer using high-dose bolus interleukin-2. *JAMA* 271: 907–913.

Royal R E, Steinberg S M, Krouse R S, et al. (1996) Correlates of response to IL-2 therapy in patients treated for metastatic renal cancer and melanoma. *Cancer J Sci Am* 2: 91–98.

Schmitz N, Linch D C, Dreger P, et al. (1996) Randomised trial of filgrastim-mobilised peripheral blood progenitor cell transplantation versus bone marrow transplantation in lymphoma patients. *Lancet* 347: 353–357.

Schrader J W (1994) Interleukin-3. In: Thomson A, ed. *The Cytokine Handbook*, 2nd edn. London: Academic Press, 81–98.

Schultz M Z, Buzaid A C, Poo W J (1997) A phase II study of interferon alpha-2b with dacarbazine, carmustine, cisplatin and tamoxifen in metastatic melanoma. *Melanoma Res* 7: 147–151.

Sheffield R E, Sullivan S D, Satiel E, et al. (1997) Cost comparison of recombinant human erythropoietin and blood transfusion in cancer chemotherapy-induced anaemia. *Ann Pharmacother* 31: 15–22.

Soiffer R J, Murray C, Cochran K, et al. (1992) Clinical and immunological effects of prolonged infusion of low dose recombinant IL-2 after autologous and T cell depleted allogeneic BMT. *Blood* 79: 517–526.

Solal-Celiggny P, Lepage E, Brousse N, et al. (1993) Recombinant interferon alfa-2b combined with a regimen containing doxorubicin in patients with advanced follicular lymphoma. *N Engl J Med* 329: 1608–1614.

Sosman J A, Fisher S G, Kefer C, et al. (1994) A phase I trial of continuous infusion interleukin-4 alone and following interleukin-2 in cancer patients. *Ann Oncol* 5: 447–452.

Sosman J A, Aronson F R, Sznol M, et al. (1997) Concurrent phase I trials of intravenous interleukin-6 in solid tumor patients: reversible dose-limiting neurological toxicity. *Clin Cancer Res* 3: 39–46.

Tamm I, Grimme H, Bergen E, et al. (1997) Dacarbazine and interferon alpha for stage IV malignant melanoma. *Oncology* 54: 270–274.

Taneja S S, Pierce W, Figlin R, et al. (1995) Immunotherapy for renal cell carcinoma: the era of interleukin-2 based treatment. *Urology* 45: 911–924.

Tepler I, Elias L, Smith II J W, et al. (1996) A randomized placebo-controlled trial of recombinant human interleukin-11 in cancer patients with severe thrombocytopenia due to chemotherapy. *Blood* 87: 3607–3614.

Tepper R I, Coffman R L, Leder P (1992) An eosinophil-dependent mechanism for the anti-tumor effect of interleukin-4. *Science* 257: 548–551.

Thom A K, Alexander H R, Andrich M P, et al. (1995) Cytokine levels and systemic toxicity in patients undergoing isolated limb perfusion with high-dose tumor necrosis factor, interferon gamma and melphalan. *J Clin Oncol* 13: 264–273.

Triozzi P L, Kim J A, Martin E W, et al. (1995) Phase I trial of escalating doses of interleukin-1β in combination with a fixed dose of interleukin-2. *J Clin Oncol* 13: 482–489.

Troussard X, Flandrin G (1994) Hairy cell leukaemia. An update on a cohort of 93 patients treated in a single institution: effects of interferon in patients relapsing after splenectomy and in patients with or without maintenance treatment. *Leuk Lymphoma* 14 (Suppl. 1): 99–105.

Vadhan-Raj S, Kudelka A P, Garrison L, *et al.* (1994a) Effects of interleukin-1α on carboplatin-induced thrombocytopenia in patients with recurrent ovarian cancer. *J Clin Oncol* 12: 707–714.

Vadhan-Raj S, Papadopoulos N E, Burgess M A, *et al.* (1994b) Effects of PIXY321, a granulocyte–macrophage colony-stimulating factor/interleukin-3 fusion protein, on chemotherapy-induced multilineage myelosuppression in patients with sarcoma. *J Clin Oncol* 12: 715–724.

Vadhan-Raj S, Murray L J, Bueso-Ramos C, *et al.* (1997) Stimulation of megakaryocyte and platelet production by a single dose of recombinant thrombopoietin in patients with cancer. *Ann Int Med* 126: 673–681.

Veelken H, Mackensen A, Lahn M, *et al.* (1997) A phase I clinical study of autologous tumor cells plus interleukin-2 gene transfected allogeneic fibroblasts as a vaccine in patients with cancer. *Int J Cancer* 70: 269–277.

Veldhuis G J, Willemse P H B, Sleijfer D T, *et al.* (1995) Toxicity and efficacy of escalating dosages of recombinant human interleukin-6 after chemotherapy in patients with breast cancer or non small cell lung cancer. *J Clin Oncol* 13: 2585–2593.

Weaver A, Ryder D, Crowther D, *et al.* (1996) Increased numbers of long term culture initiating cells in the apheresis product of patients randomised to receive increasing doses of stem cell factor administered in combination with chemotherapy and a standard dose of G-CSF. *Blood* 88: 3323–3328.

Weiss G R, Margolin K A, Aronson F R, *et al.* (1992) A randomized phase II trial of continuous infusion of interleukin-2 or bolus injection interleukin-2 plus lymphokine-activated killer cells for advanced renal cell carcinoma. *J Clin Oncol* 10: 275–281.

West W, Schwatzberg L, Blumenchein G, *et al.* (1990) Continuous infusion interleukin-2 plus sc. interferon alpha-2b in advanced malignancy. *Proc Am Soc Clin Oncol* 9: A748.

Westin J, Rödjer S, Turesson I, *et al.* (1995) Interferon alfa-2b versus no maintenance therapy during the plateau phase in multiple myeloma: a randomized study. *Br J Haematol* 89: 561–568.

Woll P J, Hodgetts J, Lomax L, *et al.* (1995) Can cytotoxic dose-intensity be increased by using granulocyte colony-stimulating factor? A randomized controlled trial of lenograstim in small cell lung cancer. *J Clin Oncol* 13: 652–659.

Yang J C, Topialin S L, Parkinson D, *et al.* (1994) Randomized comparison of high-dose and low-dose intravenous interleukin-2 for the therapy of metastatic renal cell carcinoma: an interim report. *J Clin Oncol* 12: 1572–1576.

Yin J-L, Williams B G, Arthur C K, *et al.* (1995) Interferon response in chronic myeloid leukaemia correlates with ABL/BCR expression: a preliminary study. *Br J Haematol* 89: 539–545.

11

Monoclonal antibodies as therapeutic agents

Graham R Wallace

On entering the body, a foreign substance will be met by various effector mechanisms of the immune response. One of the major mechanisms is the secretion of antibody by B lymphocytes. Antibodies are immunoglobulin (Ig) molecules with recognition sites specific for a particular structure on an antigen. Each B lymphocyte displays on its surface a unique membrane-bound immunoglobulin that functions as an antigen receptor. When a particular B lymphocyte binds antigen, it proliferates and differentiates into a plasma cell, which produces large amounts of the surface immunoglobulin in secreted form. By binding to molecules, either soluble or on the surface of organisms, antibodies label them as foreign and initiate other killing mechanisms to destroy the antigen.

Introduction to monoclonal antibodies

Antibody structure

Immunoglobulin molecules are made up of two identical light chains (MW 23 000) and two identical heavy chains (55 000–70 000). Each light chain is linked to a heavy chain by non-covalent bonds and also by a single covalent disulphide bridge. The two heavy chains are linked together by further disulphide bonds (Figure 11.1). The N-terminal half of both light chains varies greatly from molecule to molecule, whereas the C-terminal half is highly conserved. These sections are therefore classified as variable (V) regions and constant (C) regions. Likewise, in heavy chains the N-terminal section is the V region and the remainder the constant region.

There are two types of light chain, known as κ or λ chains. There are five main types of heavy chain, designated γ (IgG), α (IgA), μ (IgM),

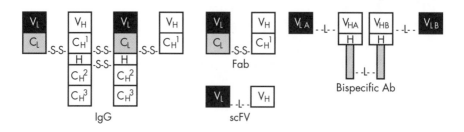

Figure 11.1 Structures of antibody molecules.

δ (IgD) and ε (IgE), and for each Ig molecule the heavy chains determine the function of the antibody. Two sets of genes control immunoglobulin synthesis, those for the light chains and those for the heavy chains. Variable region and constant region genes are separated by introns (non-coding sections of DNA), which are spliced out at the transcriptional stage to produce an mRNA that is translated into an immunoglobulin chain. Heavy and light chains are then linked by disulphide bonds to form a functional antibody molecule (Figure 11.1). Six hypervariable regions, three on the V_H (variable heavy) chain and three on the V_L (variable light) chain, combine to form the antigen recognition site known as the complementarity-determining region (CDR). It is the CDR that confers the specificity to an antibody molecule. The CDRs extend beyond the framework regions of the antibody molecules to form highly exposed domains that are able to interact with antigen. Recombination events at the time of intron splicing are responsible for most of the diversity of the antibody repertoire. The constant regions (Fc) are the effector part of the molecule that binds to components of the complement system and to specific receptors on effector cells, such as monocytes, granulocytes and natural killer cells. Functions resulting from Fc interactions include complement-mediated lysis, antibody-dependent cellular cytotoxicity, phagocytosis, cytokine production and antigen presentation. The different Fc regions elicit different functions, for instance in humans IgG1 and IgG3 are strong binders of complement whereas IgG2 and IgG4 are weak binders, therefore the isotype of the antibody is important in relation to the desired outcome. The domain structure of antibodies allows the allocation of function to particular regions and the fusion of different regions by molecular techniques to produce new molecules of given function and specificity.

Background to antibody therapy

The importance of phagocytosis in antibacterial activity was first demonstrated by Metchnikoff in 1882. In 1890, Kitasato and Von Behring demonstrated that cell-free serum from horses inoculated with toxin could protect children from disease. The first recorded case was with tetanus antitoxin, and Von Behring later demonstrated similar results with diphtheria antitoxins. These antitoxins were called antibodies. Tetanus antitoxin was used extensively during the First World War on wounded soldiers and dramatically reduced the incidence of tetanus. The opposing theories of cellular immunity, proposed by Metchnikoff, and humoral immunity (cell-free), proposed by others, were reconciled by researchers such as Sir Almroth Wright, who coined the term opsonisation to describe the binding of antibodies to bacterial surfaces, thus increasing the potency of phagocytosis by increased uptake by macrophages. Antibody-based therapies were used extensively in the early twentieth century to treat a variety of infectious diseases, including influenza, pneumonia and tetanus. The disadvantages of serum therapy, such as batch variation, inadequate dosage and a range of side-effects including fever, rash and arthralgia, collectively known as serum sickness, established the need for better therapeutic approaches.

Throughout this century, protocols for growing bacteria and viruses have allowed killed and attenuated vaccines to be derived. Moreover, the advent of sulphonamide and antibiotic drugs has greatly reduced the need for antibody therapy. However, a recent discovery heralded a new beginning for the use of antibodies. Studies of multiple myeloma cancers demonstrated that each myeloma produces antibody of a single type (i.e. monoclonal).

In 1975, Kohler and Milstein mixed mouse myeloma cells with spleen cells from an immunised mouse and produced fused cells which secreted antibody and were immortalised by the tumour cells (Figure 11.2). From this fusion they were able to select clones that secreted antibody of a single specificity that could be maintained in culture indefinitely. The clone was then injected into a mouse to produce high concentration of high-affinity antibodies of a single specificity. These

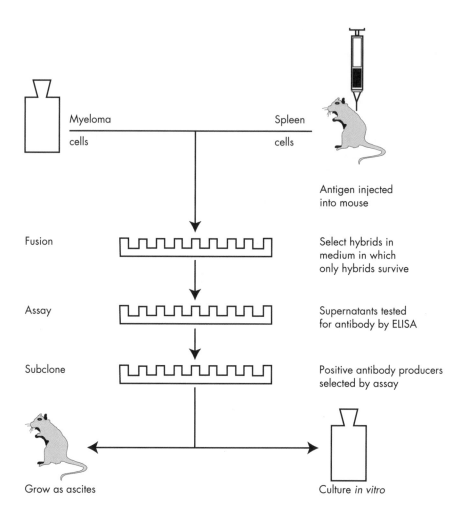

Figure 11.2 Preparation of monoclonal antibodies.

were termed monoclonal antibodies (MAbs). Compared with early serum therapy, MAbs generated by hybridoma technology or recombinant DNA techniques have all the prerequisites for a successful treatment: they are uniquely specific; they are involved in the body's defence system; they can be manipulated at the gene or protein level to alter or increase specificity; large-scale production is possible; and they are long-lived in the host. MAb-based products do not require the whole protein

– the Fab fragment, which incorporates the two CDR-binding domains, or the single-chain Fv molecule can be equally effective and in many cases desirable.

Development of monoclonal antibodies

Human anti-mouse antibodies

When monoclonal antibodies developed in the mouse are then used to treat human patients they are recognised as being foreign and a response is induced against them. Human anti-mouse antibodies (HAMAs) limit the amount of MAb reaching its appropriate target, by forming complexes with the MAb that are eliminated in the spleen, and the number of doses that can be administered to a patient. The HAMA response can also induce a form of serum sickness with fever, rash and in severe cases organ failure and fatal shock. The new technology of genetic engineering has pioneered several methods designed to overcome this problem. For example, humanisation of rodent MAbs, or indeed the large-scale production of human monoclonal antibodies, is now possible.

Humanised antibodies

The simplest type of humanised antibody is the chimaeric form, in which the antigen-specific variable regions of the mouse MAb are synthesised with the human constant regions. In this way, the recognition is still via the mouse regions, whereas the effector functions are mediated by the human portion. Moreover, much of the HAMA response is directed to the Fc region, and this is eliminated in the chimaeric molecule. Taking this idea a step further is the method of CDR grafting, in which only the rodent CDRs are transferred onto a human antibody framework. This technique is less immunogenic than the use of either parent mouse MAbs or the chimaeric form, but it has proved difficult to retain the original high affinity because amino acid residues in the human immunoglobulin alter the structure of the CDR. It has been possible to overcome this problem in some cases by computer modelling of the antibody structure and making alterations where necessary. Replacing the mouse sequence with the human sequence also increases the length of time the MAb will remain in the body: from about 1 day for fully mouse MAbs, to about 8 days for chimaeric MAbs, and up to 2–3 weeks for fully humanised

MAbs. This is important in regulating the dose of antibody and the effectiveness of the treatment.

Xenografting

A new type of hybridoma technology may play a major role in the production of human monoclonal antibodies. Human heavy- and light-chain immunoglobulin genes have been introduced into fertilised mouse embryos via a bacterial plasmid vector. Mice developed from these embryos produce functional B lymphocytes that secrete human antibodies. Transgenic technology utilises the mouse antibody affinity maturation pathways to produce high-affinity antibodies. Antibody-producing cells are isolated from the transgenic mouse and, using standard technology, fused with myeloma cells to produce a hybridoma. Fully human monoclonal antibodies can then be produced in large quantities by bioprocessors. There is no requirement to select individual genes as, by humanising the mouse, there is no need to humanise the antibody. This model is an important novel technology in raising MAbs against human antigens as it represents a naive human immune system that has not previously encountered human antigen, and therefore will produce high-affinity MAb with no tolerance induction.

Selected lymphocyte antibodies

The selected lymphocyte antibody method (SLAM) involves the isolation of antibody genes of known specificity from a single lymphocyte. Reverse transcription-PCR amplification of the V_H and V_L regions is used to produce cDNA for scFv molecules, which can then be expressed by the systems described below. This novel technology allows the selection of individual lymphocytes expressing antibodies against rare antigens and may provide a powerful technique for producing specific antibodies.

CD40 binding

Human MAbs can be produced by the stimulation of B cells via CD40. CD40 is a 45- to 50-kDa glycoprotein found on the surface of B cells, and binding of CD40 to its ligand is a requirement for B-cell activation. In this system, CD40 on the surface of the appropriate B cell, which has been immortalised by Epstein–Barr virus, is activated by anti-CD40 antibodies held on a solid support and the B cells are induced to produce antibody. Epstein–Barr virus immortalisation eliminates the need for antigen or any other cells in this system. This technology allows B lymphocytes to be maintained in long-term culture and secrete high levels of human antibody of defined specificity for therapeutic use.

Allografting

A unique approach to develop human MAbs involves infecting healthy volunteers with a vaccine directed at a known infectious agent. Polyclonal antisera are raised in these donors, from which the antibodies are then extracted and used to treat patients. Antibodies against a *Pseudomonas* protein have been developed for use in patients with cystic fibrosis, in whom bacterial problems are common.

Expression of antibody molecules

Mammalian cells

The use of recombinant DNA technology has been developed in the field of MAbs. Recombinant human antibody fragments can be expressed in a variety of systems. Inserting DNA encoding antibody genes or gene fragments, under the control of an appropriate promoter, into the desired system allows the expression and screening of the resultant product (Trill *et al.*, 1995). Mammalian cells, such as Chinese hamster ovary (CHO) cells or COS cells can produce up to 10 mg/ml depending on the DNA construct used. The benefits of this system are that mammalian cells are able to generate properly folded antibody molecules with high efficiency. Moreover, novel methods using cell types adapted for serum-free conditions have reduced the costs of producing antibody derivatives from mammalian cell systems.

Bacterial cells

Bacterial expression systems have advantages over mammalian systems in that they have much faster generation times, high yields and simpler cloning strategies (Ge *et al.*, 1995). However, a drawback is that the products are often misassembled, lack proper glycosylation (which may be important for antibody function), and may require further manipulation to produce functional protein.

Phage antibodies

MAb fragments can also now be displayed as fusion protein on the surface of filamentous bacteriophages, allowing selection of the appropriate antigen-binding activity by screening with antigen. Phage antibodies can be developed directly from the human donor, do not require immunisation of laboratory animals and can be grown in culture to produce high yields and specificity (Mark, 1995). However, as phage antibodies are produced from naive immunoglobulin genes and phage do not have the machinery for affinity maturation, phage antibodies were initially of relatively low affinity. Modification of variable regions of these molecules by site-directed mutagenesis has produced much higher affinity antibodies that show much greater binding and retention characteristics.

The second drawback with phage antibodies is the lack of Fc regions to recruit biological effector functions. This has been addressed in recent work with bispecific molecules. These so-called diabodies are antibody fragments consisting of two light chains and two heavy chains held together by linker molecules; thus the two arms of the antibody molecule can be engineered to have different specificities. Diabodies with one arm specific for a defined antigen and the other specific for immunoglobulin itself have been demonstrated to adopt the characteristics of immunoglobulin, with increased half-life and complement fixation. Other potential possibilities for this technology include one arm specific for particular Fc receptors, thereby targeting effector cells to the site, or recognition of T-cell surface molecules to attract cytotoxic cells to the site. This ability to couple biological effector processes with target antigen specificity promises to be a major advance in the use of antibodies as therapeutic reagents.

Insect cells

Expression of antibody genes in insect cells via the baculovirus system has shown promising results (Potter *et al.*, 1995). As insect cells have the ability to perform most of the complex post-translational modifications required, the resultant protein has been demonstrated to have similar functional activity to antibody molecules produced by mammalian cells. Insect cell expression systems also produce up to 10-fold higher levels of antibody derivatives than mammalian cells. New vectors that place the foreign gene in the optimum configuration, leading to increased production of the antibody protein, may increase this even further. This technology produces rapid and efficient expression of antibody proteins and may therefore be an important source of therapeutic antibody molecules.

Plant antibodies

A recent novel approach to antibody production has been the expression of intact molecules from plants (Ma *et al.*, 1995). Genes encoding IgA molecules inserted into tobacco plants produced stably assembled IgA, raising the prospect that therapeutic antibodies could be delivered directly in food. Such a method would eliminate the necessity of purifying antibody molecules and have the added bonus of directing IgA molecules to the gastrointestinal tract, where they are most effective. One possible disadvantage of this system is that the glycosylation pattern of plant-derived antibody molecules is different from that of those produced by mammalian systems, which may induce an anti-antibody response or may affect function.

Purification of monoclonal antibodies

Having been produced, purification of monoclonal antibodies is the next hurdle. There are several procedures currently available, each with strengths and weaknesses in different areas such as economy, yield and reproducibility. Each monoclonal antibody must be treated as an individual protein. Two antibodies, even if they are of the same isotype and grown in the same cell line, will have different optimal purification requirements. The standard method of purification is still precipitation, particularly for smaller amounts of antibody. Precipitation with ammonium salts is a cheap but basic procedure that lacks consistency and produces low yield. Ammonium salts are not good at clearing viruses or DNA. Other methods, including precipitation with polyethylene glycol-conjugated caprylic acid or ethacridine, are alternatives to ammonium salts but have the same problems. However, when coupled with anion-exchange chromatography, precipitation provides reasonably pure monoclonal antibody for laboratory purposes.

Protein A affinity chromatography is a popular procedure for monoclonal purification. On the plus side, this single-step technique gives up to 90% yield and has excellent clearance of contaminants such as DNA and viruses. On the down side, protein A affinity varies with different antibody subclasses, and direct protein A–antibody interactions and harsh elution conditions can alter the activity of the purified antibody.

Ceramic macroporous hydroxyapatite particles and metal affinity chromatography are new methods which are currently being used for monoclonal purification. Hydroxyapatite has a strong selectivity for immunoglobulin and metal affinity which binds to histidine-rich regions on the conserved domains of all mammalian IgG; both have high capture efficiency and elution requires only mild treatment. Such purification procedures can be incorporated into a fluidised bed support in which the MAb-containing medium is passed through the particles; while contaminants pass straight through, the antibody is retained. These methods are able to purify large quantities of antibody from bioreactors with working volumes of 500–2000 litres and, with a minimum of four purification steps, the final yield is around 60%. If MAbs are to be used routinely in therapeutic form then the technology of purification must progress with the development of the antibodies themselves.

Clinical uses of monoclonal antibodies

MAbs may be used to interfere with a variety of cellular functions. For example, activation of cells via surface receptors can induce cytokines, hormones, complement and other physiological mediators. Conversely, cells may be inactivated by monoclonal antibodies via blocking of functional receptors, ion channels or adhesion molecules.

Adhesion molecules

Adhesion molecules are families of proteins, such as selectins and integrins, which are expressed on the surface of cells and, through binding to specific ligands, link cells together. These interactions are important in lymphocyte activation, antibody production and for the binding of cells to vascular surfaces prior to tissue extravasation required in the immune surveillance of tissues. In animal models of autoimmune disease, MAbs against adhesion molecules have proved successful. MAbs against the integrin intercellular adhesion molecule-1 (ICAM-1) prevent the induction of collagen-induced arthritis in mice; likewise, anti-very late antigen-4 (VLA-4) blocks development of experimental autoimmune encephalomyelitis. Based on such information, MAbs against cell adhesion molecules are now being tested in human studies. An anti-leukointegrin HuF2G, a humanised MAb, is in phase II trials in haemorrhagic shock but may also be useful in multiple sclerosis, ischaemic stroke and heart attacks. ICAM-3, which has been implicated in signalling between lymphocytes, has been targeted in psoriasis, graft versus host disease and transplant rejection.

Cell activation markers

Autoimmune disease is caused by a breakdown in the tolerance that the immune system normally displays to self components. MAbs have the ability to regenerate antigen-specific tolerance, ameliorating the pathogenesis of these conditions. Antibodies against CD4, a molecule found on a subset of T lymphocytes, have been demonstrated to prevent a variety of autoimmune disease models in animals, such as diabetes, arthritis and systemic lupus erythematosus. Such MAbs have also proved clinically effective in the treatment of rheumatoid arthritis patients (Cobbold *et al.*, 1996).

CAMPATH-1, a monoclonal antibody that recognises Cw52, a molecule found on lymphocytes and monocytes, has been successfully employed in therapy. Inoculation of CAMPATH-1 leads to rapid lymphocyte depletion, mainly of CD4$^+$ cells. Numbers do rise again partially, but remain low. Patients treated with CAMPATH-1 still have decreased CD4$^+$ cell counts up to 2 years after therapy. In rheumatoid patients, swollen joints and morning stiffness are alleviated and most patients report feeling better on this treatment compared with conventional protocols, and those who are also on disease-modifying drugs respond better. Small numbers of patients remain in remission, while others relapse. CAMPATH-1 has also been tested in vasculitis patients and has proved successful with remissions of up to 4 years (Lockwood *et al.*, 1996). In multiple sclerosis patients, CAMPATH-1 significantly decreases the number of neurological lesions detected by magnetic resonance imaging. In seven patients, a total of 79 lesions were detected prior to treatment, 15 in the 3 months following treatment and only two in the next 3-month period.

MAbs against specific T lymphocyte antigen-binding receptors, which recognise autoantigens, have been successfully tested in animal studies, inhibiting arthritis and neurological disease. The identification of specific TCR usage in human disease may pave the way for similar treatment.

The induction of tolerance is also very important in preventing graft rejection. Antibodies against a variety of T lymphocyte surface markers, such as CD3, CD25 and CD28, have been used to induce tolerance to grafts. Blocking of T-cell surface molecules inhibits the induction of T-cell activation and so enhances graft survival. Several MAbs have been proven effective in clinical trials. OKT3, an antibody that binds to the epsilon chain of the CD3 molecule, has been shown to inhibit graft rejection in kidney transplant patients. Possibly one of the most successful therapies may be to combine MAbs against CD4 and CD8, which are found on different subsets of T lymphocytes. In animal experiments, this protocol has been demonstrated to block graft rejection and induce long-term tolerance in recipient animals given mismatched tissue. These experiments strongly suggest that induction of long-term tolerance in humans may be possible with non-lytic MAbs (i.e. antibodies that do not induce cell destruction) and immunosuppressive drugs together to redirect the immune response from an aggressive to a suppressive state (Scully *et al.*, 1997).

Unmodified antibodies recognising particular structures on cell surfaces have also been effective in tumour therapy. Single chain Fv molecules (Figure 11.1) that recognise the immunoglobulin idiotype (formed by the CDR of antibody) expressed on B-cell lymphoma cells have been developed for use as vaccines. When inoculated into the host, a response is raised against the idiotype region and the resultant antibodies recognise not only the ScFv molecule but the immunoglobulin on the lymphoma cell surface, thereby directing effector mechanisms to these cells.

An alternative to targeting the cells involved in pathogenesis directly is to block the mediators that signal between them. Recent studies with a MAb against TNF have proved beneficial in patients with rheumatoid arthritis, with a reduction in both clinical and laboratory parameters of disease in both low dose (11/25 patients) and high dose (19/24) compared with patients on placebo treatment (2/24) (Elliott *et al.*, 1994). A larger trial of this treatment is now under way.

Immunotoxins

Paul Erlich, the German bacteriologist, first coined the term 'magic bullet' to describe a compound that is selectively toxic to a specific target. Erlich's research was aimed at discovering chemical compounds with this characteristic, whereas modern-day magic bullets include immunotoxins which have toxic moieties bound to antibody and immunoconjugates which have radionuclides attached to the MAb.

MAbs developed against tumour-associated antigens have been developed and subsequently linked to either radionuclides or poisons. The antibody molecule provides the specific targeting element directing the killing moiety to the correct cells. The most widely used is the plant toxin ricin, which consists of two linked polypeptide chains, A and B, which bind to galactose residues on cell-surface molecules via the B chain. Following endocytosis into the cytosol, the A chain interacts with the ribosome pathway leading to cell death. Because of the non-specific nature of the B-chain binding, ricin is used in the form of the A chain alone or both ricin A and ricin B but with the galactose binding sites blocked.

The diphtheria toxin acts in a similar manner to ricin, with its B chain binding to an epidermal growth factor (EGF) receptor and, once inside the cell, the A chain acting on the same stage of the ribosome pathway. A truncated form of diphtheria toxin (DAB486) that lacks the EGF receptor has also been developed to prevent non-specific binding. A bacterial exotoxin from *Pseudomonas* (PE) binds to cells via the α_2-macroglobulin receptor and kills by a similar mechanism to diphtheria toxin.

Immunotoxins have been tested in several clinical trials in cancer patients. Ricin linked to anti-CD5, a marker on T cells and some B cells, has been used in T-cell lymphoma and B-cell chronic lymphocytic leukaemia. Similarly, ricin linked to anti-CD19, a B-lymphocyte marker, has been tested in patients with non-Hodgkin's lymphoma. In experimental animal models, PE40, a truncated form of the *Pseudomonas* toxin comprising the A chain only, and DAB486, linked to monoclonal antibodies against the IL-2 receptor expressed on activated T lymphocytes, have been demonstrated to block allograft rejection.

Radionuclides attached to MAbs that recognise the IL-2 receptor have also been used as therapeutic agents. Anti-IL-2 receptor antibody coupled to yttrium-90 has been used in clinical trials of patients with leukaemia with good results, and in 2/17 cases complete remission was achieved.

To obtain greater efficiency, the different elements can be introduced separately. Pre-targeting involves the injection of antibody–avidin complex, which labels the target cells. Avidin, a glycoprotein present in egg white, is composed of four subunits that form a tertiary structure with four biotin (vitamin H) binding pockets. The radionuclide or toxin, attached to biotin, is then introduced and either binds to the cell-bound antibody via avidin or is rapidly cleared from the body. This technique increases the specificity of the killing and decreases bystander targeting, hence identifying only those cells carrying the markers recognised by antibody.

Animal models have demonstrated the use of secondary compounds to increase the efficacy of immunoconjugates. The cytokines IL-1β and GM-CSF, given either as a bolus or by continuous infusion, lead to an increase in the tolerated dose of some radioconjugated MAbs. Moreover, preinfusion with the radiosensitisation agent bromo-deoxyuridine prior to treatment with an ^{131}I-labelled MAb causes a dramatic reduction in tumour size in animals.

Coupling a cytotoxic drug, DM1, a very potent anti-cancer agent, to the monoclonal C242, which binds to a protein on colon tumour cells, has given interesting results in trials. It was found that this combination eliminated tumours in mice, whereas antibody or drug alone had little effect. The combination therapy also showed minimal toxicity in this animal model.

A chimaeric monoclonal, C2B8, which targets the CD20 molecules on B lymphocytes and tumour B cells in non-Hodgkin's lymphoma has shown a 50% response rate in a trial of 190 patients, 70% of whom were still in remission at 10 months. The effectiveness rose to 100% when C2B8 was used in conjunction with conventional chemotherapy. C2B8 acts by stimulating the body's normal defences, such as complement, to attack tumour cells and therefore does not require conjugation to a toxic agent. The benefit of this monoclonal is that CD20 is not expressed on B-cell precursors and B-cell levels recover to normal in a few months.

Immunotoxins have been shown to be effective in several types of tumours, however solid tumours are still very difficult to treat owing to the inability of the immunotoxin to penetrate the tumour mass. This may improve with the development of ScFv fragments produced by bacterial systems, which are smaller, and therefore should enter more easily into the target tissue.

Another novel approach to targeting solid tumours is Techniclone's tumour necrosis therapy (TNT), which uses a MAb carrying a toxic payload to the inner core of tumours. Cancer cells, unlike normal tissue, undergo rapid degeneration, resulting in areas of necrosis (dead tissue) at the tumour centre, where the cell membranes become leaky, allowing large molecules such as antibodies to enter the cell. In TNT, the MAb binds to DNA, which only becomes accessible in dead or dying cells; upon attachment it delivers the toxic moiety inside the cell, destroying the tumour from inside out.

A recent development in increasing the specific effectiveness of immunotoxins has been to fuse the antibody molecule to a DNA-binding protein that is bound to a plasmid containing the toxin gene. This construct produces a molecule that is relatively stable and non-toxic compared with direct conjugation with the toxin protein. The MAb directs the binding of the fusion molecule to the target cell, and only after the complex is internalised and the plasmid becomes operational will production of the toxin begin. This method reduces non-specific damage that may occur when immunotoxins are used. Expression can be made even more selective by placing the toxin gene under cell-specific promoters, which will only induce toxin gene expression in the appropriate cell.

Recent advances in directing toxins to the tumour site or cell and reducing toxic side-effects of these potent molecules will increase the use and effectiveness of immunotoxins as therapeutic agents.

Imaging

An important use for MAbs, labelled with radionuclides, is the visualisation of tumours without the need for exploratory surgery. The specificity of the MAb directs the label to the site, which can then be pinpointed by radioimmunodetection. This technique has now been used in several different studies. An MAb labelled with indium-111 has been used to detect intra-abdominal metastases that have been missed by computerised tomography (CT) scans. An $F(ab)_2$ MAb against carcinoembryonic antigen (CEA) labelled with iodine-131 identified relapse in colorectal cancer patients with an 86% accuracy. Moreover, a Fab fragment to the same antigen but labelled with technetium-99 identified metastases in 70% of patients whose tumours could not be detected by conventional imaging. Similarly, a ^{99}Tc-labelled MAb against a B-cell lymphoma antigen imaged additional tumour sites in 30% of non-Hodgkin's lymphoma patients tested. This method has also been used in identifying colorectal and small cell lung carcinomas. Imaging has proved to be effective post heart attack to detect dead cardiac muscle and also to visualise blood clots. This enables clinicians to evaluate the extent of the damage and to prevent further attacks due to blood clots.

In a recent study, diagnostic imaging for colorectal cancer using a humanised MAb against tumour cells linked to ^{99}Tc was tested against CT in pre-surgery patients. The presence of tumour was confirmed by surgery. The predictive value of the MAb was 60% compared with 29% for CT and had only 4% false positives.

One aspect of tumour biology that can be used in detection is angiogenesis, the growth of new vessels. Fibronectin is a large glycoprotein that is involved in cell migration and angiogenesis and is highly expressed in tumour tissue. A MAb against fibronectin detects primary and secondary lesions in 60% of patients with different forms of tumour.

Imaging is proving a very successful application of MAb technology, and as more tumour-specific antigens are identified and higher affinity human antibodies are developed this procedure will continue to be an important tool in cancer treatment.

Immunoadhesins

Immunoadhesins are designed with a region from a receptor or an adhesion molecule replacing the light chains and the V_H regions. The fusion protein is generated by ligated cDNA molecules, which are then expressed in mammalian cell systems or insect cells. Immunoadhesins can be purified in the same manner as MAbs from culture supernatant. The Fc region of the fusion protein confers specific effector functions and increases the half-life of the adhesin region by evading clearance via the kidney. The adhesin used can determine the function of the fusion protein. If a receptor molecule is fused to the Fc region, then such molecules can be used in targeting effector function to specific cells. Immunoadhesins have also been effectively used to identify ligands on the surface of cells. A third role for these molecules, neutralisation of cellular mediators, is the most advanced. In particular, immunoadhesins based on receptors for the proinflammatory cytokine TNF have been shown to be effective in animal models of rheumatoid arthritis, multiple sclerosis and uveitis (Ashkenazi and Chamow, 1997). In human trials in patients with sepsis, who produce large amounts of TNF, the results have been confusing. In the most advanced stages of disease, the TNF immunoadhesin was not effective in preventing mortality, whereas at less advanced stages of sepsis some benefit was seen. The dosage and form of the immunoadhesin, i.e. which of the two TNF receptors was used, were thought to be crucially important. A phase III trial is now under way using a TNF receptor 1-IgG molecule, based on these initial findings.

Although not strictly MAbs, immunoadhesins that direct effector responses to specific cells or neutralise pathogenic molecules may prove to be useful in autoimmune and inflammatory conditions, and transplantation involving blocking surface molecules on invading cells may lead to graft acceptance.

Table 11.1 Clinical trials in progress

Trial	Disease	Number
Recognition of surface markers	Cancer – lymphoma, leukaemia Sepsis Autoimmune disease HIV Transplantation	54
Immunotoxins	Leukaemia Small cell lung cancer Colorectal cancer	11
Imaging	Liver Breast Cardiovascular thrombosis	15

Conclusions

Monoclonal antibodies have made a major impact on several areas of biological science. As specific markers for cell-surface molecules, they have been used for identification, separation of cells and killing. For soluble molecules such as protein antigens, MAbs have been invaluable in purification techniques and allow sufficient quantities to be collected and analysed. Currently, 80 monoclonal antibodies are in clinical development, making them the largest category of all new therapeutics being tested by the biotechnology industry (Table 11.1). The techniques described in this chapter for humanising MAb will provide high-affinity antibodies that will not be recognised as foreign, and in future MAb-based therapy will be at the forefront of medical science.

Acknowledgements

I would like to thank Carolyn Watson for producing the figures and Brian Ellis for helpful discussions on the manuscript.

References

Ashkenazi A, Chamow S (1997) Immunoadhesins as research tools and therapeutic agents. *Curr Opin Immunol* 9: 195–200.
Cobbold S P, Adams E, Marshall S E, *et al.*(1996) Mechanisms of peripheral tolerance

and suppression induced by monoclonal antibodies to CD4 and CD8. *Immunol Rev* 149: 5–33.

Elliott M J, Maini R N, Feldmann M, *et al.* (1994) Randomised double blind comparison of chimaeric monoclonal antibody to tumour necrosis factor alpha (CA2) versus placebo in rheumatoid arthritis. *Lancet* 344: 1105–1110.

Ge L, Knappick A, Pack P, *et al.* (1995). Expressing antibodies in *Escherichia coli*. In: Borrebaeck C A K, ed. *Antibody Engineering: a Practical Guide*, 2nd edn. Oxford: Oxford University Press, 229–243.

Kohler G, Milstein C (1975) Continuous cultures of fused cells secreting antibody of predefined specificity. *Nature* 256(5517): 495–497.

Lockwood C M, Thiru S, Stewart S, *et al.* (1996) Treatment of refractory Wegener's granulomatosis with humanised monoclonal antibodies. *Q J Med* 89: 903–912.

Ma J K C, Hiatt A, Hein M, *et al.* (1995) Generation and assembly of secretory antibodies in plants. *Science* 268: 716–719.

Mark J D (1995) Human monoclonal antibodies from V-gene repertoires expressed on bacteriophage. In: Borrebaeck C A K, ed. *Antibody Engineering: a Practical Guide*, 2nd edn. Oxford: Oxford University Press, 53–69.

Metchnikoff E (1884) Ueber eine Sprosspilzkrankheit der Daphnien. Beitrag zur Lehre uber den Kampf der Phagcyten gegan Krankheitserreger. *Arch. fur Pathologische Anatomie und Physologie und fur Klinische Medicin.* 96: 177–195.

Potter K N, Li Y C, Capra J D (1995) Antibody production in insect cells. *ACS Symposium Series* 604: 41–55.

Scully R, Cobbold S P, Mellor A L, *et al.* (1997) A role for Th2 cytokines in the suppression of CD8 T cell mediated graft rejection. *Eur J Immunol* 27: 1663–1670.

Trill J J, Shatzman A R, Ganguly S (1995) Production of monoclonal antibodies in COS and CHO cells. *Curr Opin Biotechnol* 6: 553–560.

Von Behring E, Kitasato S (1890) Ueber das Zustandekommen der Diphtherie-Immunitat und der Tetanus-Immunitat bei Thieren. *Deutsche Med Wochenschrift* 16: 1113–1114.

Glossary

Adhesion molecule   Protein that mediates binding of one cell to another or to the extracellular matrix.

Adjuvant   Substance that enhances the immune response to an antigen with which it is mixed.

Allele   An alternative form of a gene. Alleles of a specific gene occupy the same location on homologous chromosomes. Thus, in a diploid cell, each gene will have two alleles, each occupying the same position on homologous chromosomes.

Altered peptide ligands   Peptides in which one or more of the amino acids in the 'native' peptide has been substituted for another amino acid.

Annealing   The process whereby DNA sequences combine by hydrogen bonding with other complementary sequences as temperatures fall below a critical denaturation or melting temperature.

Antibody   Immunoglobulin molecule, produced by B lymphocytes, with recognition sites specific for a particular structure on an antigen.

Antigen   A molecule that reacts with an antibody to stimulate T cells.

Antigen presentation   Process whereby antigens – usually fragments of proteins – are displayed on the surface of a cell together with molecules (MHC) required for lymphocyte activation.

Antisense RNA   A sequence of RNA that is the base pair complement of an mRNA. Binding of the antisense RNA to the mRNA (also referred to as the sense RNA) blocks translation of the mRNA into protein.

Autoimmune disease   An immune response to self antigens that induces tissue damage and disease.

Bacteriophage   Double-stranded DNA viruses that infect bacteria.

Base pairing   The specific association of nucleotides to each other by hydrogen bonding. In DNA, adenine (A) pairs with thymine (T) and guanine (G) pairs with cytosine (C). In RNA, adenine (A) pairs with uracil (U) and guanine (G) pairs with cytosine (C).

Blastocyst   The spherical, cohesive group of 8–16 cells formed after the first three or four divisions of the zygote.

cDNA library   A complete copy of all the genes expressed in a particular cell type in the form of cDNA.

CentiMorgan (cM)   A measure of the genetic distance between two linked marker genes on a chromosome. For example, 1 cM is equivalent to 1000 kb at the nucleotide level.

Chromosome   A strand of tightly compacted DNA containing sequences of DNA (genes) encoding for proteins and their regulation of expression. Chromosomes are present in all cells. In mammals (including humans), all chromosomes are paired except for the sex chromosomes.

Codon   Part of the genetic code. A sequence of three nucleotides in an RNA molecule that encodes for an amino acid. Many amino acids make up a protein.

Complementary DNA (cDNA)   Artificially produced copy of mRNA. Used because of its increased stability compared with mRNA.

Copy number   Number of replications of the DNA sequence.

Cytokines   Proteins produced by cells that affect the action of immune cells.

Deletion   Loss of a region of genomic DNA from a chromosome that results in the loss of part of a gene or of a number of genes which can generate pleiotropic phenotypes.

Denaturation   The process whereby double-stranded DNA is heated to a temperature at which the hydrogen bonds between complementary DNA strands break to give two single strands of DNA.

DNA   Deoxyribonucleic acid.

DNA-dependent DNA polymerase   An enzyme that will add nucleotides to the $3'$ end of a DNA strand that already is bound to a complementary DNA strand but which has single-stranded DNA to act as a template.

DNA fingerprinting   A technique to identify DNA sequences that are specific to an individual. The technique involves restriction enzyme digestion of genomic DNA followed by Southern blotting to detect minisatellite regions in the DNA that are specific for a specific individual's genetic make-up.

DNA replication   The process by which cells copy their genomic DNA before cell division.

Dominant mutation   Mutation in one gene copy (allele) resulting in expression of a disease phenotype.

Duplication   Gain of a region of genomic DNA in a chromosome that results in the duplication of a part of a gene or of a number of genes that can generate pleiotropic phenotypes.

Effector T cells   Cells that can remove pathogens from the body.

Epitope   Site on an antigen that stimulates the immune system.

ES cells   Embryonal stem cells. Established in tissue culture from explanted blastocysts.

Exon   Region of DNA that is found in the mature mRNA. Derived from the term 'expressing sequence', exons can be divided into coding and non-coding exons. Coding exons contain sequence that codes for amino acids, whereas noncoding exons contain sequence that is found in the untranslated regions of the mRNA. The number of exons in specific genes can vary from 1 to more than 20.

Founder animal   Animal that has been developed from an injected egg.

Fv (variable fragment)   Variable region/antigen-binding domain of an antibody molecule.

Gene   A sequence of nucleotides that encodes for a protein and its expression in the cell.

Genetic linkage   Genes or DNA markers at two or more loci are inherited together as a result of their close proximity on a chromosome. When they are physically close together the linkage is said to be tighter and there is less chance that they will be separated during meiosis.

Genome   The total genetic content of a cell.

Genotype   The genetic constitution of an individual cell or organism.

Germ cell Sperm, egg or early embryo.

Helicase The enzyme that disrupts the secondary structure of double-stranded DNA to produce single-stranded DNA so that DNA replication can occur.

Homologous genes Genes that give rise to proteins with similar function but which have different protein sequences. Often a gene in two related organisms will have the same function but a slightly different sequence and is said to be homologous.

Homologous recombination Genetic recombination that occurs between DNAs with long stretches of homology (e.g. between homologous chromosomes at meiosis) and which is mediated by enzymes that show no particular sequence specificity. Homologous recombination can be used to target introduced DNA to particular regions of the chromosome, thus disrupting selected genes.

Idiotype Antigen binding site of the immunoglobulin expressed on the surface membrane of tumour cells.

Immunoblotting (Western blotting) Technique of identifying specific proteins following electrophoretic resolution, transfer and immobilisation to a membrane support and incubation with a specific antibody.

Infection (with a retrovirus or adenovirus) A method of inserting a therapeutic gene into a recipient cell.

Intron The region(s) of DNA that do not code for gene products and which are removed during the generation of mRNA. Derived from the term 'intervening sequences', introns are found between the exons of a gene and are sometimes referred to as 'junk DNA' because of the apparent lack of biological function. The number of introns in specific genes can vary from 0 to more than 20.

Isoforms Genes or proteins with similar, but not identical, sequences that can have different functions found in the same organism and often in the same cell.

Karyotype The full set of chromosomes of a cell arranged with respect to size, shape and number.

Knockout The process of preventing the expression and function of a protein by introducing a DNA sequence that will inhibit translation of the messenger RNA encoding the gene.

Locus The position or location of a gene (or a gene polymorphism) on a given chromosome.

Major histocompatibility complex (MHC) Cluster of genes encoding for molecules that are able to present antigens to lymphocytes.

Messenger RNA (mRNA) An RNA molecule that carries the message for protein synthesis.

Minisatellite DNA A short sequence of DNA that consists of a tandem repeat. These sequences are known to occur in regions of DNA that vary greatly between individuals and are used as the basis of an individual's DNA fingerprint.

Monogenic disorder A disease caused by a single-gene defect.

Multiple-locus probes DNA fingerprinting probes that have sequence similarity with many repeat regions in the genome and so recognise multiple bands on a Southern blot of genomic DNA and give rise to the classical DNA fingerprint pattern.

Northern blotting Technique of identifying specific RNA sequences following electrophoretic resolution, transfer and immobilisation to a membrane support and hybridisation with a specific labelled probe.

Nucleotide An organic molecule containing a purine (adenine or guanine) or pyrimidine (thymine or cytosine) base, a five-carbon ribose or deoxyribose sugar and one or more phosphate groups.

Nucleotide triphosphate A nucleotide with three phosphate groups which is the building block of DNA and the energy source for many chemical reactions.

Oligodendrocyte Cell responsible for producing central nervous system myelin.

Oligonucleotide A short sequence of nucleotides (usually fewer than 30).

Peptide Short fragment of a protein comprising a number (usually fewer than 20) amino acids.

Phenotype The observable character of a cell or organism.

Plasmid Circularised DNA fragment distinct from genomic DNA, isolated from bacteria, used as a cloning vector.

Polymerase chain reaction (PCR) The technique whereby small quantities of specific sequences of DNA can be amplified exponentially to provide analytical quantities of DNA.

Polymorphism A difference in DNA sequence between individuals. This may give rise to alterations in gene function and can be found in both introns and exons. Polymorphisms are useful for linkage analysis and can be associated with specific diseases and populations.

Primer A short sequence of DNA or RNA (up to 30 bases) used to prime the elongation of DNA replication.

Primer, degenerate A mixture of DNA oligonucleotides that vary only by one or two bases.

Promoter Region of the gene that signals the initiation of transcription (i.e. copying of mRNA from DNA).

Pronucleus The nucleus of either the unfertilised egg or sperm.

Pseudopregnant female A female in oestrus that has been mated with a vasectomised or genetically sterile male.

Recessive mutation Mutation of both alleles of a gene causing the phenotype to be expressed.

Replicon Sequence in the DNA that initiates replication.

Reporter gene A marker gene that is easy to detect once transfected into cells, e.g. β-galactosidase, which produces a characteristic blue colour in those cells that have taken up the gene. Used to study the levels and efficiency of expression of the transfected gene.

Restriction enzyme Enzymes that cut (digest) DNA at specific sequences.

Ribozymes RNA molecules that possess enzymatic activity and have potential as therapeutic agents as they can cleave mRNA molecules or affect the repair of mutant RNAs.

RNA Ribonucleic acid.

RNA primase An enzyme that lays down a 10-base strand of RNA using single-stranded DNA as a template.

Sequence The order of nucleotides or amino acids found along a strand of DNA or a protein, respectively.

Short tandem repeat polymorphisms (STRPs) Small repetitive nucleotide sequences that exist in tandem arrays of varying repeat numbers.

Single-locus probes Highly specific repetitive element probes that recognise a single repeat element in genomic DNA. Southern blots probed with a single-locus probe generate two distinct bands and give rise to a DNA profile rather than a DNA fingerprint.

Somatic cell   All cells except germ cells.

Southern blotting   Technique of identifying specific regions of DNA following restriction enzyme digestion, electrophoretic resolution, transfer and immobilisation to a membrane support and hybridisation with a specific labelled probe.

Sticky ends   Protruding, cohesive 5′ termini that are produced in DNA strands cut with certain restriction enzymes.

Stringency   The degree of selectivity used to anneal a DNA sequence to its complementary strand, decided either by temperature or by buffer composition.

Taq **polymerase**   A heat-stable version of DNA-dependent DNA polymerase obtained from the bacterium *Thermus aquaticus*.

T-cell receptor   Cell surface-related molecule on T lymphocytes that recognises peptide antigen in association with an MHC molecule.

Transduction   The transfer of non-viral DNA by a virus into a cell.

Transfection   The insertion of genes into cells (mammalian).

Transformation   The insertion of genes into cells (bacterial).

Transgene   The foreign DNA that is transferred to and expressed in the recipient animal.

Transgenic   The introduction of a gene from one species into the germ line of another distantly related species.

Vector   A circular self-replicating DNA molecule into which the gene of interest is inserted prior to transfection into mammalian cells or transformation into bacteria.

Western blotting (see Immunoblotting)

Xenotransplantation   The transfer of an organ or cell from one species to another, unrelated species.

Zygote   A fertilised egg.

Index